MALIGNANT

Medical Ethicists Confront Cancer

Edited by
Rebecca Dresser

D0171167

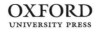

OXFORD
UNIVERSITY PRESS

OXFORD
UNIVERSITY PRESS

Oxford University Press, Inc., publishes works that further
Oxford University's objective of excellence
in research, scholarship, and education.

Oxford New York
Auckland   Cape Town   Dar es Salaam   Hong Kong   Karachi
Kuala Lumpur   Madrid   Melbourne   Mexico City   Nairobi
New Delhi   Shanghai   Taipei   Toronto

With offices in
Argentina   Austria   Brazil   Chile   Czech Republic   France   Greece
Guatemala   Hungary   Italy   Japan   Poland   Portugal   Singapore
South Korea   Switzerland   Thailand   Turkey   Ukraine   Vietnam

Published by Oxford University Press, Inc.
198 Madison Avenue, New York, New York 10016

www.oup.com

Oxford is a registered trademark of Oxford University Press

Library of Congress Cataloging-in-Publication Data

Malignant : medical ethicists confront cancer / edited by Rebecca Dresser.
      p. ; cm.
       ISBN 978-0-19-975784-8
    1. Cancer—Popular works. 2. Cancer—Patients—Care—Moral and ethical aspects.
              3. Caregivers—Psychology. I. Dresser, Rebecca.
    [DNLM: 1. Ethics, Medical—Autobiography. 2. Neoplasms—diagnosis—Autobiography.
3. Caregivers—psychology—Autobiography. 4. Neoplasms—psychology—Autobiography. QZ 201]
                   RC263.M32 2012
        174.2'96994—dc23   2011015612

1 3 5 7 9 8 6 4 2

Printed in the United States of America
on acid-free paper

Malignant

For the families, friends, doctors, and nurses
who helped us through cancer

Contents

Preface

This book tells the stories of seven people who are all too familiar with cancer. Once upon a time, our knowledge of cancer was mainly academic. Before cancer became a personal matter, most of us had worked for years in the medical ethics field (Arthur Frank went into ethics after having cancer, but before that taught medical sociology). We read and talked about cancer because it was relevant to what we taught at our universities and medical schools. That changed when we were diagnosed with cancer, or learned that a husband or wife had cancer. At that point, we really began to learn about cancer.

In one of our group discussions, Patricia Marshall referred to "a strange duality" in cancer: While you are suffering through what you hope will be life-saving treatment, you see death "standing outside the window, looking in." This particular duality is one many cancer patients and their loved ones experience, but the people in our group experienced a second strange duality. This was a duality between the professional and personal.

The professional–personal duality pervaded our cancer experiences. Some of us had cancer treatment in the same places we taught and worked. One month, we were parking in the hospital lot on our way to teach medical students; the next month, we were parking in that same lot on our way to have surgery or chemotherapy. One month, we were sitting next to a colleague at an academic meeting; the next month, we were asking that colleague to help us find a good cancer surgeon. One month, we were reviewing cancer study proposals as members of research ethics committees; the next month, we were considering whether to sign up for one of those studies.

The professional–personal duality didn't end when treatment ended. Today, when we bump into our doctors at work or walk past the chemotherapy center on the way to a lecture, we are transported back to the time when we were sick and vulnerable. When we open a medical journal to read an ethics article, we come across studies reporting treatment results for people with the same types of cancer we dealt with. Where we once would have ignored these reports, we now can't resist reading them—they illuminate our futures and remind us of lost loved ones. These are the queasy moments, the times when "professional cancer" becomes "personal cancer."

At first, not everyone in our group was enthusiastic about writing a book. Some were reluctant to climb onto the cancer bandwagon. Not so many years ago, cancer was something people didn't talk about. Today, it seems the opposite is true. Cancer memoirs are everywhere, along with news stories, movies, plays, television shows, and novels about cancer. In one of his chapters, Art Frank mentions a woman who feels she has "failed Cancer 101," because she hasn't written a book. With so many people talking and writing about their cancer experiences, some of us wondered whether we had anything new or useful to contribute to the cancer literature.

Some also hesitated because they did not want to, as John Robertson put it, "get back into the world of cancer." They asked the questions we all asked at some point during this project: Now that we have (we hope) gotten through the worst part of cancer, why revisit those awful days? Cancer takes up more than enough of our psychic energy as it is—why take on something that will require us to obsess about it even more? The office is a place to get away from cancer and focus on other things, but now you are asking us to think about cancer there, too?

But truthfully, we weren't able to escape cancer at the office. Whether we liked it or not, close encounters with cancer were an occupational hazard. As medical ethics professors, we couldn't avoid coming across cancer. Since we couldn't escape cancer at home or at work, we decided to dive in, hoping we could bridge the gap between our personal and professional understandings. It also seemed urgent to relay what we had learned, in the hope that it might ease the way for future patients and their families.

Like most people who have been through cancer, we were shocked by the experience. In telling our stories, we hope to help others avoid at least some of the painful surprises. We also believe that the dominant public picture of cancer is incomplete. It may seem as though everyone dealing with cancer has to talk, write, or somehow make public the experience, but this isn't true. Plenty of people want to get as far away as possible from cancer, and plenty fear that cancer will overwhelm everything else in their lives. Plenty feel stigmatized, and plenty feel abandoned because no one around them wants to recognize that cancer is in the room.

Plenty of patients and families are downcast and depressed, too. Public messages about winning wars and racing for cures don't have much to do with the actual lives of most people dealing with cancer. Patients and families more often feel like civilians in an unwinnable war—overmatched by the enemy and at risk from the friendly fire of chemotherapy and other harsh treatments.

So, we wanted to try to bring together our two types of cancer knowledge, and we thought we could provide a less upbeat, more heterogeneous picture of what it can mean to have cancer. In the pages that follow, we take what we learned as patients and caregivers, and show how it fits—or does not fit—into medical ethics. We consider the conventional understanding of issues like patient decision-making and point out deficiencies in that understanding. More often, we find problems that medical ethics has ignored, or at least neglected. In the midst of serious illness, people are helped and harmed in a number of ways that haven't captured the attention of people in our field.

We wrote this book for three groups. We wrote for patients and their families, hoping to alert them to some of the problems they may face. We wrote for doctors and nurses, hoping to show them what ethics looks like from the perspective of cancer patients and their caregivers. And we wrote for our colleagues, because what we learned belongs in the medical ethics conversation.

We know we haven't begun to cover everything about ethics and personal experience with cancer. There is much more to say about each topic we consider, and there are lots of important topics we didn't get to. We know, too, that people will disagree with what we write, or have experiences that differ from the ones we describe. We hope that they will speak up about this, and will supply the information and insights we missed. We want this to be the start of a conversation, not the final word.

We have many people to thank. The following people read and commented on chapter drafts: Douglas Adkins, Steve Joffe, Peter Joy, Mary Grace Kessler, Helen Kornblum, Janice Loomis Romond, Ann Davis Shields, Alan Wertheimer, and Rebecca Dresser's Washington University Law School colleagues. The Greenwall Foundation provided financial support, and its president, Bill Stubing, cheered us on.

Peter Ohlin was enthusiastic and understanding as we worked to pull the manuscript together. Rebecca Dresser also received research support from Washington University Law School. Jamie Roggen and other faculty assistants at Washington University Law School put in long hours preparing the transcripts of our meetings. Kristen Schwendinger provided valuable research assistance.

We will donate all royalties from this book to organizations assisting cancer patients and their families.

Rebecca Dresser
St. Louis
February 2011

Contributors

Dan W. Brock is the Frances Glessner Lee Professor of Medical Ethics in the Department of Social Medicine and Director of the Division of Medical Ethics at the Harvard Medical School. He served as staff philosopher on the President's Commission for the Study of Ethical Problems in Medicine and was a member of the Ethics Working Group of the Clinton Task Force on National Health Reform.

Rebecca Dresser is the Daniel Noyes Kirby Professor of Law and Professor of Ethics in Medicine at Washington University in St. Louis, where she teaches medical and law students about issues in bioethics. She is the author of *When Science Offers Salvation: Patient Advocacy and Research Ethics*. From 2002 to 2009, she served on the President's Council on Bioethics.

Norman Fost is Professor of Pediatrics and Bioethics and Director of the Bioethics Program at the University of Wisconsin. He has been Chair of the Hospital Ethics Committee for 25 years and was Chair of the Health Sciences research ethics board for 31 years. He has served on numerous federal advisory groups, including the Clinton Task Force on National Health Reform.

Arthur W. Frank is professor of sociology at the University of Calgary. His first book, *At the Will of the Body*, is the story of his own illnesses. It won the annual writers' award from the U.S. National Coalition for Cancer Survivorship. Another one of his books, *The Renewal of Generosity*, won the 2008 annual medal in bioethics from the Royal Society of Canada.

Leon R. Kass is the Addie Clark Harding Professor Emeritus in the Committee on Social Thought at the University of Chicago, and Hertog Fellow at the American Enterprise Institute. From 2001 to 2005, Kass served two terms as chairman of the President's Council on Bioethics. In May 2009, he delivered the Jefferson Lecture for the National Endowment for the Humanities.

Patricia A. Marshall is professor in the Department of Bioethics, Case Western Reserve University School of Medicine. A medical anthropologist, her work focuses on cultural diversity and bioethics practices. She has been a consultant to the National Bioethics Advisory Commission and the World Health Organization's Council for International Organizations of Medical Sciences.

John A. Robertson holds the Vinson & Elkins Chair at The University of Texas School of Law at Austin. He is the author of *The Rights of the Critically Ill* and *Children of Choice: Freedom and the New Reproductive Technologies*. He is a fellow of the Hastings Center and past chair of the Ethics Committee of the American Society for Reproductive Medicine.

Malignant

CHAPTER I

Crash Course

Rebecca Dresser

Sometimes it seems that cancer is everywhere you look. In nearly every family, someone has had cancer. Everyone knows someone who has had this disease. Women in the United States have just over a one in three chance of having cancer and men nearly a one in two chance. Cancer causes one in four deaths in this country, and it's estimated that more than 11 million living Americans have a history of cancer.[1] About 40% of Americans will get cancer sometime during their lives, and their loved ones will be intimately affected, often as caregivers.

How should we respond to cancer's massive presence? What we hear most often is that we must find a cure. Above all, we are told, we must create a world without cancer. The only meaningful response to cancer is to eradicate it.

Yet, cancer probably cannot be eradicated. Pledges "to eliminate . . . suffering and death from cancer"[2] are misleading, more a product of wishful thinking than realistic appraisal. In our lifetimes and beyond, cancer will continue to be a common disease and a leading cause of death in countries rich enough to keep threats like malnutrition and infectious disease at bay. Cancer will continue to make huge demands on the doctors, nurses, and other clinicians who look after seriously ill patients.

It's certain that many of us, as well as the people we know and love, will confront life-threatening cancer. Cancer will force itself into our lives, and we will be called upon to respond as persons, as individuals. Yet, most of us are ill-prepared for that event.

No one teaches us how to respond to cancer, but respond we must. One place to turn to for guidance is the stories of those who have already been face to face with cancer. Personal stories make cancer real; they create authentic portraits of cancer to counter simplistic public images of this disease. Patients and their families can tell others what to expect when cancer intrudes and how to get through the ordeal. Learning about the experiences of others is a way to prepare for cancer in our own lives.

This book tells the cancer stories of seven people who work in the field of medical ethics. Five of us have had cancer, and three have cared for spouses with cancer (one has been both a cancer patient and caregiver). In these pages, we describe what we learned from our experiences—what helped us, harmed us, surprised us, and humbled us.

We bring both bad and good news from the cancer front. Cancer hits people hard, transforming the lives of patients and the people who care for them. A cancer diagnosis brings with it sudden and unwelcome immersion in the medical system. Drastic treatment measures usually follow, disrupting ordinary home and work life. Relationships with doctors and nurses come to the forefront. Mortality is no longer something in the background that is easy to ignore.

Much of the cancer experience is bleak. This is true even for privileged people like us. We had good health insurance coverage and medical colleagues we could call on for advice and support. Even with these advantages, navigating the health care system was tough. With cancer, you become dependent on overworked doctors and nurses who often can't give you the attention you need. You wait what seems like too long for everything, and you wait with other patients desperate for the same care that you require. Sometimes, though, the system works wonderfully. You are rescued by kind and sensitive clinicians whose capacities amaze you. You appreciate in a new way the doctors and nurses who surmount the obstacles to become true members of the healing professions.

The nonmedical part of the cancer experience has dark and bright sides, too. Cancer reminds healthy people of their vulnerability to illness and death, and this affects how they behave toward patients and caregivers. Some people seem gifted with "perfect pitch," able to give comfort and support in just the right ways. Others are uneasy and don't know what to say or do. Some people make things worse by talking about the wonderful vacation they have planned for the week you are scheduled to start chemotherapy or the incredible spiritual growth that will come from your "cancer journey." Some people see your cancer as their own personal tragedy, and you find yourself comforting them, instead of the reverse.

Much of what happened to us will happen to others. Cancer is different for each individual, but there are also plenty of shared experiences. In writing about our encounters, we hope to help others prepare for cancer. We think our stories will also be useful to clinicians seeking to make cancer care better and to medical ethicists seeking to make the field more relevant to patients and caregivers. By examining ethical issues through the lens of the cancer experience, we seek to expand and enrich existing ethical thinking about cancer, as well as to extend and deepen the general understanding of this terrifying, yet quite common, disease.

THE WAY WE LOOK AT CANCER

Before cancer entered our lives, most of us had worked for years in the medical ethics field. You might think that a background in medical ethics is good preparation for dealing with cancer. We are not so sure about that. It's true that we knew more about the medical system than most patients do. We were used to reading medical journals and participating in medical meetings, so we knew how to talk to doctors and find out more about our cancer and its treatment. Because of our work, we knew doctors who could help us with treatment decisions and come to our aid when the system broke down. Knowing these things was helpful, but we didn't feel ready for cancer. Although some of us had an easier time than others, cancer wasn't easy for any of us.

We did not feel particularly prepared for cancer, but we did have a certain frame of reference for the cancer experience. Before cancer became a personal matter, we were used to thinking about serious illness from an academic, professional perspective. We had discussed cases involving cancer patients with medical students, doctors and nurses, and hospital ethics committees. Cancer was embedded in many of the topics we examined in our teaching and writing, topics like end-of-life care and medical research.

This background affected our perceptions of cancer, making us particularly alert to matters of ethics. When doctors told us about the cancer diagnosis, we were frightened in the same way that anyone is when cancer is announced. At another level, however, we were watching the way the message was delivered. Our doctors were "breaking bad news," a subject we had encountered in medical ethics teaching and scholarship. We had studied truth-telling about serious illness and now we were seeing it done. We heard the unwelcome announcement primarily as patients and caregivers, but we also heard it as medical ethicists. The ethical gaze we had developed through our work was still in operation.

In short, we came to cancer with a certain perspective. Our training became the context for our personal experiences with cancer. Our backgrounds led us to see the ethical dimensions of our interactions and to test our experiences against what we had read, written, and taught about serious illness. We don't claim to possess unusual wisdom about the cancer experience, but we do have a distinct outlook on what happened to us.

WHAT WE LEARNED

Although we had a particular way of looking at cancer, we quickly discovered we were not experts in real-world cancer ethics. We found that our ideas about patient autonomy were too abstract, too cerebral. Making treatment decisions was more difficult than we had expected, and we were surprised at how much we depended on doctors to help us make treatment choices. The rights and wrongs of caring for cancer patients were not always as clear as we had previously believed.

We discovered as well that we had inaccurate preconceptions about cancer. Cancer is far from a unitary disease. Cancer can mean death, but it can also mean long-term survival. Cancer can be the worst sickness imaginable, or it can be less terrifying than other medical conditions. Cancer treatment can involve multiple rounds of onerous chemotherapy, or one relatively simple surgery. Cancer can impose drastic life changes or small-scale adjustments in ordinary routines. We learned that there is much variation in the cancer experience.

We found ethics in unexpected places, too. Cancer patients and caregivers may spend lots of time in treatment centers and doctors' offices, but they spend much more time in the outside world. Many of our most significant interactions were with people we knew from our pre-cancer lives. But not everyone knows how to talk with friends and colleagues facing life-threatening illness. Because cancer makes people uncomfortable, they may turn away or make thoughtless remarks to patients and their caregivers. We don't claim to have learned exactly the right things to say, but we do have examples of helpful and hurtful exchanges. Our experiences showed us that ethical thinking about cancer belongs in everyday life, as well as in medical settings.

Personal experience also alerted us to the individual moral challenges cancer presents. Cancer is a forceful reminder that life is finite. Existential questions like "How should I live?" and "What do I care about most?" suddenly loom large. Cancer patients and caregivers confront loss of control, vulnerability, and increased dependence. Hope and denial become necessities, but so do realism and honesty about treatment trade-offs and the losses that cancer can bring. The future becomes less clear than it seemed before, and judgments about an acceptable quality of life can change. Cancer can bring loneliness, isolation, and depression, but it can also bring renewed intensity to life.

After cancer, "everything is different and nothing is different."[3] Cancer brought us face to face with our mortality, but our mortality was there all along. Cancer changed us physically and psychologically, but much about us remains unchanged. Cancer was a personal crisis, but it is only part of who we are. Cancer left us acutely aware of life's blessings, but we still take too much for granted. We continue to examine what we can and should make of our cancer experiences and the life that remains.

Our experiences led us to realize that cancer ethics is not just a medical concern. As a result, in these pages we write not only about matters widely identified as "official" medical ethics topics, such as breaking bad news and treatment decision-making, but also about what might be called "hidden" ethics topics, such as cancer stereotypes and survivor responsibilities. Our stories involve not only doctors and other clinicians, but also relatives, friends, colleagues, students, and others we encountered during our time as patients and caregivers. We describe not only what cancer taught us about medical care, but also what cancer taught us about ourselves—about, for example, our unrealistic desires for independence and control. In drawing attention to topics like these, we seek to expand customary notions of medical ethics, to go beyond ethics in the medical setting to ethics in the social and personal worlds of serious illness.

OUR STORYTELLING APPROACH

Cases and stories make common appearances in medical ethics, for real events capture audiences in ways that abstract analysis cannot. People in medical ethics recognize that presenting illness stories is an effective way to engage students and readers. But relatively few medical ethicists use their own cases as the basis for professional work. Telling stories about other people is different from telling your own stories.

In telling our stories, we join a long line of individuals who have written powerfully about personal experiences with cancer. Memoirs by people like Reynolds Price, David Rieff, and Marjorie Williams[4] helped us to make sense of our own situations. We owe a great debt to these storytellers, and we don't suggest that we can improve on their work. But we do have a different focus. We put ethics at the forefront, offering systematic and fine-grained ethical analysis not included in other personal accounts. We tell our personal stories, but then we consider them from our professional vantage points.

This book also differs from other cancer stories because it brings together a group. Although one person's experience may be reasonably representative of what others go through, one person can never capture the variety of cancer experiences. Our experiences and responses to cancer are diverse, and our stories reflect that. We dealt with different types of cancer, different prognoses, and different treatment regimens. Three of us have faced serious health problems in addition to cancer. Two classify their cancer experience as less disturbing and demanding than their experiences with other illnesses, but one has the opposite view.

Our differences go beyond the medical. We are individuals with different personality styles and dispositions. Our personal values, family situations, and life histories are different, too. Although we all work in the medical ethics field, we have different educational backgrounds, including medicine, law, sociology, anthropology, and philosophy. Six of us had long careers in medical ethics before becoming cancer patients or caregivers, but one of us had cancer before going into the field. Because we are different in these and other ways, our perspectives on cancer are different. We have different cancer stories and different opinions on what implications to draw from those stories. In these pages, we compare, contrast, and disagree about various dimensions of the cancer experience.

Our stories describe the way things seemed to us. We realize that there are other ways of looking at the same events. Some people who were part of our stories reviewed our accounts and helped with details and accuracy. But we recognize that we don't have access to the full truth of what happened to us. Our stories were also written after the fact, when we could be more thoughtful about events that were confusing and chaotic at the time. Some of us kept illness journals that helped us recapture our earlier impressions. But memories are imperfect, and what we describe in retrospect might not be exactly the description we would have given in real time. We think storytelling is a good way, not a flawless way, to explore the ethics of serious illness.

Serious illness is an intimate matter, and we reveal a good deal of ourselves in our stories. Without self-revelation, our stories would be less authentic and less instructive. We have tried to protect the privacy of the other characters in our stories. The living individuals we name have given us permission to do so. We believe the loved ones lost to cancer would approve what we have written. We don't identify most of the people in our stories, including the doctors and nurses who cared for us. Some individuals involved in our care generously reviewed draft materials and supplied useful feedback on what we had written.

HOW WE BEGAN

A cancer story explains how we came to write this book. During cancer treatment, many patients feel rotten. I was one of them. Reading and watching television helped pass the time, but it was often hard to concentrate. I spent hours not feeling well enough to work or read even low-brow mysteries. In an attempt to battle the boredom, I kept the radio on and paid attention when I could.

One day as I was drifting between sleep and wakefulness, I heard a reporter talking with two doctors who had been diagnosed with cancer after years of experience caring for patients.[5] Through becoming cancer patients, they said, they had learned a lot about how to practice medicine. I realized that I felt the same way about my experience. Since my diagnosis, I had been immersed in a crash course in real-world medical ethics. Having cancer was horrible, but I was fascinated by the world I had entered. I was learning so much about ethics from the patient's point of view, and I wanted to put that new knowledge to use.

News spreads quickly when you have cancer. You hear from lots of people and from a surprising number of them, you hear personal stories of cancer. Some of the personal stories I heard came from colleagues in medical ethics. Once I was back on my feet, I told these colleagues about my idea and asked if they would like to join a project I was calling "Cancer and Bioethics: When the Professional Becomes Personal." Six people said they would like to participate, so I put together a proposal and secured funding for the project.

When we gathered to talk about cancer and ethics, it was a different sort of meeting for us, one with an unusually personal cast. We talked about ourselves in unaccustomed ways. We felt the strong bond that comes from sharing an intense personal experience. There was much more emotion than usual.

Yet, there was plenty of analysis at our meetings, too. We considered our experiences in the context of our medical ethics training. Our cancer stories resembled the cases we were used to examining in our ethics work, only this time we had a different kind of understanding of what had happened. Our discussion mixed personal, subjective accounts with the objective approach we customarily applied to medical cases. As you might expect with a group of professors, we argued about how to interpret our stories and what lessons to take from them. We taped and transcribed our conversations. The transcript, together with personal essays we wrote before each meeting, became the raw material for this book.[6]

Our meetings covered three stages in the typical patient's life: diagnosis, treatment, and life after treatment. We talked about our experiences with misdiagnosis and conflicting medical opinions. We exchanged stories about telling loved ones and others of the diagnosis. We assessed the pros and cons of being open about our situations and gave examples of responses that did and did not help us through this intense and unsettled period. We talked about what it was like to step away from our jobs and other commitments so that we could deal with the demands of cancer treatment.

We also discussed what life was like during and after surgery, chemotherapy, and radiation therapy. We described the burdens treatment imposed, how we coped with them, and points at which they became overwhelming. We talked about side effects, changes in appearance, and restrictions on ordinary activities. We told stories about incidents in the hospital and encounters with medical students, residents, and cancer center volunteers. We examined interactions with other patients, including those who served as our "cancer mentors." We discussed what we did to preserve connections to people in the world beyond home and treatment center.

As we reviewed our experiences, we considered how a number of general concepts come into play for cancer patients and caregivers. These concepts make frequent appearances in medical ethics. Some apply to the patient–doctor relationship. They include truth-telling, breaking bad news, trust, professional boundaries, patient autonomy, medical paternalism, informed consent, confidentiality and "hanging crepe" (a strategy doctors have of presenting the worst-case scenario to patients and families so that they will be prepared if it materializes, and pleasantly surprised if it does not).[7] Clinicians are often advised to respect "the patient as person,"[8] and we examined the meaning of this ethical aspiration in the medical setting.

A collection of concepts with ethical significance in both the medical setting and the wider social world also came up in our discussion. These concepts include dignity, privacy, empathy, compassion, stigma, and fairness. And, as we considered our individual responses to cancer, concepts like hope, denial, guilt, grief, and redemption made frequent appearances. These ideas and ideals were part of the ethical backdrop as we analyzed our stories.

SPECIFIC CANCER MATTERS

Our conversations became the foundation for this book. The chapters that follow examine thirteen specific topics that engaged our group. Eight chapters focus on medical experiences, three on attitudes and interactions outside the medical setting, and two on cancer's personal moral impact. Chapters draw heavily on the record of our group discussion and on the individual essays we prepared before each of our meetings. Chapters emphasize the experiences of their authors, but also include stories and reflections from others in the group.

"Diagnostic Quests and Accidents" considers initial symptoms, tests, and examinations preceding the cancer diagnosis. Some of us were diagnosed with late-stage disease after our symptoms were overlooked or dismissed. Those in this category wonder how much to blame physicians for failing to detect cancer earlier, and how much to blame themselves for failing to take symptoms more seriously. Others in our group were diagnosed promptly after cancer screening or annual physical examinations, and one is alive because a clinician treating a separate medical problem ordered an unnecessary test that detected cancer at an easily treatable stage. These individuals are grateful that their cancers were discovered sooner rather than later, but their gratitude is mixed with a recognition that luck and privilege had a lot to do with it. This chapter examines how clinical competence, personal behavior, privilege, and fortuity can affect when cancer is diagnosed.

"Learning the Bad News" describes how we learned of the cancer diagnosis. No doctor enjoys telling patients that they have cancer, but many doctors must take on this painful chore. Although some of our doctors performed the task with honesty and sensitivity, others did not. A few tried to pass the responsibility to others. Some didn't seem to appreciate the impact their message would have on us. And even when physicians performed admirably, we were devastated by the announcement. There is no good way to hear that you have cancer, but there are better and worse ways. This chapter discusses what was helpful and harmful in this situation, and offers our thoughts on what clinicians can do to comfort and support patients confronting life-threatening illness.

"Coping with Uncertainty" describes what it was like to decide among treatment options with uncertain outcomes. In choosing a treatment approach, we were gambling with our lives. Some of us "took charge" of our cases, using the Internet and professional contacts to inform our treatment choices. Others relied primarily on personal physicians to explain what we needed to know about treatment alternatives. Sometimes it was easy to see which treatment regimen was most likely to succeed, but often the evidence was unclear. Sometimes what our doctors said about treatment outcomes was different from the statistics we read elsewhere. We wanted certainty, but knew that was impossible. All we could do was hope to be one of the lucky ones who survive cancer and its treatment relatively intact. This chapter discusses how patients and doctors manage the unavoidable uncertainties that come with cancer and its treatment.

"Autonomy and Persuasion" also considers cancer treatment choices, but with a different emphasis. This chapter examines how personal values and circumstances shaped our decisions to accept or refuse medical interventions. A variety of factors influenced our treatment choices, not always for the better. We found that making good choices wasn't always easy. Our medical ethics background didn't completely shield us from irrational decision-making. We learned that conversation and argument may be needed to dissuade patients from ill-considered decisions. This chapter discusses the complexities of personal choice and challenges conventional notions of how patients exercise autonomy in the context of serious illness.

"Volunteering for Research" reports on our experiences with clinical trials. Although some of us were willing to join studies involving data collection about treatment outcomes and side effects, none of us enrolled in a trial comparing different treatments for our disease. I had the opportunity to participate in such a trial, but declined. I did so because I believed that trial participation was not in my personal best interests. Yet, the medical treatment I received was available only because previous cancer patients had been willing to participate in trials like the one I refused to join. Was my decision ethical? This chapter discusses whether patients have a duty to volunteer for research, how physicians should present research options to patients, and what patients should (but often fail to) understand about trial enrollment.

"Resilience and the Art of Living in Remission" describes what happens once cancer treatment is finished. Several of us have become members of what Art Frank once named "the remission society."[9] Although we have returned to jobs and other activities, some of us are hampered by the aftereffects of cancer or its treatment. Our cancer appears to be gone, but we face years of medical monitoring to detect signs of a recurrence or new cancer. We wonder about the benefits and harms of all the monitoring and resent cancer's continuing power over our lives. We approach the scans and examinations with trepidation, knowing the results could once again turn our lives upside down. With close scrutiny of our bodies come suspicious findings that usually turn out to be nothing serious. But even false alarms take a toll, for the wait between the finding and the reassurance is almost unbearable. This chapter describes life on the remission roller coaster and the ethical challenges it presents for patients, caregivers, and clinicians.

"The Allure of Questionable-Benefit Treatment" considers last-resort measures, such as cancer therapies that extend life for only a few patients. Two members of our group lost spouses to cancer. In both cases, doctors were willing to try treatments that had a remote chance of extending life. One patient decided to "go for it" and the other declined because the odds against success seemed too great. In both cases, patients, caregivers, and doctors found it difficult to forgo one last effort at treatment. Our cancer experiences taught us how strong the desire for survival can be. But we also know that last-resort measures can inflict damage on patients and families. Unlike some patient advocacy groups, we see real problems with making such measures widely available. This chapter describes those problems and considers how doctors can help patients and caregivers make realistic decisions about questionable-benefit interventions.

"Cancer Stereotypes" examines ways in which our experiences both reinforce and contradict various cancer stereotypes. Our cancer experiences were similar in some respects, but quite different in others. Having cancer was "not that big a deal" for two people in our group. For them, cancer involved a single surgery and relatively good survival prospects. Indeed, these individuals have other medical problems that present more significant threats to their well-being and survival.

For the rest of the group, cancer was a much bigger deal. Some of us suffered through burdensome and debilitating treatment regimens that offered less reassuring survival odds. And two of us cared for spouses as they died of cancer. This chapter describes features that do and do not set cancer apart from other serious conditions and considers whether cancer deserves its status as the "Dread Disease."[10] The chapter also considers whether cancer's public image distorts attitudes toward cancer patients and contributes to ethically questionable policies governing cancer medicine and research.

"Caregivers, Patients, and Clinicians" examines the demands put on spouses and others who take on the caregiver role. Cancer's impact on relationships can be immense. Couples must adjust to significant changes in everyday roles and activities. Caregivers must put aside work and other personal projects to help patients manage medical matters. Caregivers feel responsible for protecting their loved ones from treatment burdens, and guilty when they are unable to do so. Although clinicians usually welcome caregiver involvement, some resent it when caregivers speak up for patients. Patients preoccupied with their own miseries may take caregivers for granted, or blame caregivers when the medical system doesn't work as it should. Caregivers must walk a fine line between supporting the patient and speaking up when the patient is being careless or foolish. Yet, something of lasting value can come from these experiences, for going through the ordeal often brings people closer together. This chapter considers the many ways that caregivers sustain patients during and after cancer treatment.

"Cancer Interactions: Caring Well and Caring Badly" looks at how people responded to our cancer news. None of us tried to hide this news. Although most of us generally keep quiet about our personal lives, we found it impossible to keep quiet about cancer. This openness brought rewards, for people often reached out in magnificent ways. But this wasn't always so. We heard plenty of annoying cancer advice, as well as tales of other people's relatively minor health scares. A surprising number of people were silent, presumably at a loss for words or frightened by the reminder that they could easily be in our situation. This chapter describes what it was like to be on the receiving end of this behavior and presents our views on how people can give meaningful support to cancer patients and caregivers.

"Support, Advocacy, and the Selves of People with Cancer" presents the bright and dark sides of groups that offer support to and advocate on behalf of people with cancer. As cancer patients and caregivers, we have mixed feelings about these groups. We recognize that support groups offer great comfort, but also think they can put pressure on patients to conform to the "cheerful warrior" model. We value advocates' efforts to show the human face of cancer and raise money for patients lacking access to good care. But we think campaigns to "cure cancer" promote false hope and distract from the needs of the many patients whose cancer cannot be cured. This chapter examines the role of support and advocacy groups and their positive and negative effects on the people they endeavor to serve.

"Cancer and Mortality: Making Time Count" describes how the cancer experience affects a person's perceptions of life and the future. Cancer is a brutal reminder that human life is finite. Abstract knowledge that death is inevitable becomes painfully real when cancer is diagnosed. Couples confront the reality that they will not always be together. Sometimes they must say goodbye to each other, a task for which no one can prepare. Those who have witnessed the death of a spouse know that the unthinkable can happen. Those in remission know that death will never again appear as distant as it once seemed. But cancer also intensifies appreciation for the life that remains. And it can prepare people for the decline that at some point comes to nearly everyone who survives into the later decades. This chapter describes the sorrow and wisdom that come with cancer's teachings on mortality.

"Survivorship: In Every Expression a Crack" considers how those fortunate enough to survive cancer make sense of the experience. Once cancer is (at least temporarily) in the background, people become members of what Albert Schweitzer called, "the Fellowship of those who bear the Mark of Pain."[11] For most people, life will be different after cancer, but in what way will it be different? Survivors can look to different models of survivorship, but each person must decide how to accommodate the new knowledge cancer has conferred. The patients in our group are grateful to be alive and most feel the pull to "give back" in some way. Group members who were caregivers feel moved to reach out to others, too. Indeed, this book emerged out of our desire to help others facing cancer. But we are still uncertain about what sorts of cancer survivors we want to be. None of us, not even the one who has survived for over twenty years, has it completely figured out.

"Last Words" sums up and presents general themes. It explains why this book is relevant to medical ethics and describes how personal accounts of illness can add value to ethical analysis. It examines small-scale medical ethics: the everyday actions that express respect and concern, or disrespect and callousness, toward cancer patients and their families. It discusses how individual variation among patients complicates the clinician's task. It concludes by describing how cancer altered our thinking about medical care and about life. It presents ideas for improving patient care and social responses to cancer, but acknowledges that burdens and distress are unavoidable. There are better and worse ways to respond to cancer, but no one escapes from it unscathed.

Notes

1. These figures exclude noninvasive cancers and basal and squamous cell skin cancers. American Cancer Society, *Cancer Facts & Figures 2010*. Retrieved January 18, 2011, from http://www.cancer.org
2. In 2003, the director of the National Cancer Institute announced that his agency intended to achieve this goal by 2015. Jocelyn Kaiser, "After Regime Change at the National Cancer Institute," *Science* 312 (2006): 357–59.
3. Leon Kass uses this phrase in his chapter, "Cancer and Mortality: Making Time Count."
4. Reynolds Price, *A Whole New Life* (New York: Scribner, 2003); David Rieff, *Swimming in a Sea of Death: A Son's Memoir* (New York: Simon & Schuster, 2008); Marjorie Williams, "Hit by Lightning: A Cancer Memoir," in *The Woman at the Washington Zoo: Writings on Politics, Family, and Fate*, ed. Timothy Noah (New York: PublicAffairs, 2005), 307–39.
5. Joanne Silberner, *When Physicians Get Cancer* (National Public Radio Broadcast, April 6, 2006). Retrieved January 18, 2011, from http://www.npr.org/templates/story/story.php?storyID=5326183
6. Because the essays and transcripts contain highly personal material, we have agreed to keep these documents confidential.
7. See Mark Siegler, "Pascal's Wager and the Hanging of Crepe," *New England Journal of Medicine* 293 (1975): 853–57.
8. This phrase comes from the classic medical ethics book, Paul Ramsey, *The Patient as Person: Explorations in Medical Ethics* (New Haven: Yale University Press, 1973, 2nd ed. 2002).
9. Arthur W. Frank, *At the Will of the Body: Reflections on Illness* (Boston: Houghton Mifflin, 1991, 2nd ed., 2002), p. 138.
10. This phrase comes from James Patterson, *The Dread Disease: Cancer and American Culture* (Cambridge: Harvard University Press, 1987).
11. Quoted by Arthur W. Frank, *The Renewal of Generosity: Illness, Medicine, and How to Live* (Chicago: University of Chicago Press, 2004), p. 55.

CHAPTER 2

Diagnostic Quests and Accidents

Norman Fost

P atients take different paths to the cancer diagnosis. Some are diagnosed after consulting doctors about what turn out to be symptoms of cancer. Some are diagnosed as a result of cancer screening or routine checkups. Some are diagnosed in the course of tests or treatment for an entirely different medical problem. Our cancer and ethics group includes individuals who took each of these diagnostic paths.

As we learned, clinician competence and patient psychology often determine when cancer is diagnosed. When patients and clinicians fail to take symptoms seriously, the diagnosis comes late and the cancer is harder to treat. On the other hand, early diagnosis can lead to debilitating treatment that might be medically unwarranted. And, as I discovered, diagnosis can be a fluke—a consequence of an unjustified medical intervention that unexpectedly reveals cancer. This sort of fortuitous discovery saves some patients' lives. But it comes at a cost that even I, one of those incredibly lucky patients, cannot defend.

THE ACCIDENTAL SURVIVOR: IT'S BETTER TO BE LUCKY THAN GOOD

I have dodged four bullets in the last decade: four different life-threatening diagnoses, three of them discovered through medically unnecessary and unwarranted tests. Three of my illnesses involved life-threatening tumors—cells gone wild. I am a beneficiary of the inefficient and wasteful American health care system that I criticize on a regular basis.

I begin with my closest encounter with cancer. In May of 2006, I had a sudden kidney stone attack. Having endured many previous attacks, I knew what lay ahead. I would have excruciating, unremitting, unimaginable pain, far above the hospital wall chart's highest score. I would have to plead first with an emergency department admissions clerk and then with a nurse to skip the ritual list of screening questions and exams and give me immediate access to intravenous narcotics. With some guilt, I would ask to bypass others waiting in the emergency room—some of them might have ailments more serious than mine, but none was likely to be in as much pain as I was. The narcotics would cause me to vomit, and drugs to control the vomiting would leave me dizzy and disoriented. Throughout the ordeal, I would be worried that the stone would not pass. If it didn't, I would have to undergo an unpleasant and painful invasive procedure to have it removed.

I was very familiar with this routine, but that didn't make it any easier to manage. When an earnest young resident said he wanted me to have a computed tomography (CT) scan, I put on my doctor hat and tried to explain that, in my view, a scan was medically unnecessary. The doctors didn't need a scan to diagnose my kidney stone—the diagnosis was obvious. The scan would show where the stone was located, but that information wouldn't change anything about my treatment. The scan itself wouldn't be painful or risky, but I was not in the mood to be taken through a maze of hospital corridors to the cold scanning room, where I would have to wait who knows how long until the scanner was available.

The resident's demand also irritated my academic sensibilities. Not only would the scan serve no medical purpose, it would be an unnecessary expense. Although my insurance would cover it, the scan would be a waste of money, money that could be used on other, more justified patient care. And, instead of supplying information that would be medically useful, the scan might yield what we call in medicine an adventitious, or incidental, finding—a possibly important medical finding unrelated to my kidney stone. Adventitious findings are often ambiguous, with uncertain medical meaning. Ambiguous findings typically lead to more tests and to anxiety for patients, but usually prove to be nothing serious. I thought the scan would do more harm than good in my case.

Yet, despite my concerns, I didn't refuse the scan. My previous illness experiences had taught me the importance of patient diplomacy. I knew that there was a delicate balance between being the compliant "good patient" that doctors favor, and being the argumentative and irritating patient they dislike. As a physician, I knew too much about the medical rights and wrongs in my treatment, and as a professor, I was often tempted to lecture to the young doctors tending to me. But this time I resisted temptation, limiting myself to a brief argument about why the scan wasn't justified. I decided to save my bullets for the more important fights that might lie ahead, and agreed to be rolled away to the scan room.

As I expected, the scan was of no help in managing the kidney stone, which mercifully passed over the ensuing week. And, as I expected, there was an adventitious finding: a four-centimeter mass on the upper part of my right kidney. But, as I had *not* expected, there was little ambiguity about the meaning of the finding: It was almost certainly kidney cancer.

I learned this only after I returned home from the emergency room and got a disturbing telephone call from the radiology technician. He asked me to come back because the radiologist had seen something unusual on the scan. I immediately thought it might be cancer, so it was a tense drive back to the hospital. I drove carefully, because of something that had happened years ago in my medical practice. A man's newborn baby was dying in the hospital, and I didn't want to give him the bad news over the telephone. I called and asked him to come in right away. But he knew something was wrong. He was upset and drove recklessly, killing a teenager on a bicycle. As John Robertson describes in the next chapter, missteps in breaking bad news aren't unusual in medicine.

When I talked with the doctor, he told me that the scan showed a tumor whose size put me on the borderline between having an excellent prognosis following surgery, and having metastatic cancer with little chance of survival. Later, the news got better. More CT scans, this time with a stronger medical rationale, uncovered no evidence of metastasis. If the surgery went well, I had an excellent chance of being cured. I spent the next few weeks trying to decide which surgical approach would be best for me. I also had to decide whether to get care from my long-standing doctor or a "superstar" in another city. In addition to the trade-offs between surgery close to home or in a strange city, I worried about offending my personal surgeon, a urologist who had provided extraordinary care throughout my long history of kidney stones.

These dilemmas paled into triviality when I learned that a dear friend and medical ethics colleague had recently died of kidney cancer, which had metastasized to his brain. Like tens of thousands of people every year, he learned about his long-silent disease only after it had spread. At the time of his diagnosis, his choices were not the relatively good ones I faced. I simply had to select from among alternatives that all had a good chance of success. My friend's only choices were about how to live his remaining time in the best way, which he did brilliantly.

If the emergency room resident hadn't insisted that I have a medically unnecessary scan, I probably would have suffered the same fate as my friend. Thanks to the scan, my fate was quite different. Several weeks later, I had an uneventful operation in my home hospital to remove part of my kidney. My most memorable complication was minor, but uncomfortable: a month of intractable constipation.

Earlier, while I lay in the emergency room bemoaning my situation, I began writing in my head an op-ed piece called "Unintelligent Design." In it, I planned to describe the utter uselessness of kidney stones and the senseless, agonizing pain they inflict. Fortunately, I never published it. The senseless stone, combined with a senseless scan, saved my life.

The kidney cancer was just one of my three lucky, but accidental, diagnoses. Within a year, I had my first inkling of another life-threatening tumor, this one in my brain. Again, it was discovered through what was probably an unnecessary imaging procedure. Nine years earlier, I had had two transient ischemia attacks, or "mini-strokes." Despite being a doctor who should have known better, I spent several months denying the possibility that the attacks signaled something serious. When I finally consulted a doctor about them, tests showed that I was in danger of having a serious stroke. The doctor prescribed a drug called Coumadin (in ordinary language, a blood thinner), and said I should have regular magnetic resonance imaging (MRI) scans and other tests to monitor the situation.

After several years of no significant change and no more mini-strokes, my wife asked me a question I often ask residents and medical colleagues: "Why are you getting all these scans?" She knew that I frequently quoted my esteemed teacher and former colleague, Dr. Lew Barness, who famously said, "Ordering a lab test is like picking your nose in public: You should know ahead of time what you're going to do with the result." I decided to put this question to my superb neurosurgeon and shyly asked why we were imaging my brain. As long as I had no symptoms, the scans wouldn't affect the management of my condition. My neurosurgeon agreed that the scans were probably no longer necessary. But then he told me that on the most recent scan, there was a tiny shadow located near the back of my brain. The shadow might not be anything medically significant, he said, or it might be a tiny meningioma—a benign and usually slow-growing tumor.

The scan that detected the shadow was arguably unnecessary, but now there was a good medical reason to continue the yearly scans. The shadow grew slowly but steadily over time, making meningioma the most likely diagnosis. When it seemed to be heading for my brainstem, my neurosurgeon became more concerned. He expected the tumor to keep growing, and thought it should be removed before it did serious damage. It would also be prudent to act soon, while I remained healthy enough to withstand the surgery and he remained healthy enough to perform it.

So, in December of 2008, I had brain surgery. The tumor was in fact not a meningioma, but something called a cavernous hemangioma—an unruly mass of tiny tangled blood vessels. While official medicine wouldn't classify it as a "malignant" tumor, to me it was definitely malignant. It was a miracle that it had never bled, as these tumors tend to do. Even a small bleed in this compressed area might have killed me instantly. It was an added miracle that it had not bled during the time I was taking two drugs—Coumadin and aspirin—that increase the risk of bleeding.

Ironically, I was quite familiar with the risks posed by my condition. My first medical publication was a report on a novel treatment for children with dangerous hemangiomas, and I had maintained a life-long professional fascination with these strange and interesting tumors. Once again, my life had been saved by an adventitious finding from an arguably unnecessary scan, a test I would probably have criticized had I heard about it at medical rounds or a teaching conference.

My third dodged bullet involved that most common of mindless medical tests—the "complete blood count," commonly known as the CBC. This test supplies information about the number and character-istics of a person's blood cells. Doctors automatically order a CBC test for nearly every patient admitted to a hospital, as well as for outpa-tients having blood drawn for almost any reason. I have had many CBC tests in my life; some were done for good reasons, but most were not.

Unlike most patients, I can understand my CBC test results. As I looked at them over the years, I noticed that the number of platelets, which are one type of blood cell, was increasing. When I thought they were getting too high, I decided it would be prudent to consult with a blood specialist. When he saw the number continuing to increase, he suggested that I might be headed toward another kind of cancer—a type of leukemia that is difficult to treat. Apart from that, the increase in platelets made my blood thicker. Thicker blood put me at risk of a major stroke, because it could clog the narrow blood vessel that had led to my earlier mini-strokes. As a preventive measure, the specialist recommended something simple: a daily pill containing a mild chemotherapy drug that can suppress the platelet count without interfering with the other blood cells. I have been taking the pills for five years now, and they have been effective. Once more, I was rescued from a potential cancer catastrophe by a probably unnecessary medical test.

In sum, I was saved three times by tests that had little to no medical justification. Because of these tests, potentially life-threatening conditions were detected early, at a treatable stage. I am extremely grateful to be alive and to have escaped most of the burdens cancer imposes on patients. Yet, my good luck also leaves me with guilty feelings. When I hear about what cancer has done to other people, I have survivor's guilt. Why am I alive and well, while others have suffered and lost loved ones?

I also have another form of guilt, something I call "hypocrite's guilt." I personally benefited from the unnecessary and expensive diagnostic testing I regularly criticize in my work as a doctor and medical ethicist. In my professional teaching and writing, I often speak out against our health care system's mindless reimbursement of medically unjustified tests and treatments that cost millions of dollars and help relatively few patients.

The point of "wasteful" health care is not that it has no value. We could save lives if we paid for everyone to have CT scans every six months, or mammograms throughout the lifespan (although, because they involve radiation and can lead to unnecessary biopsies, the tests would harm some people, too). But we can't afford to save every life that is savable. The value of human life is not infinite, and our limited resources are needed for health care that provides more bang for the buck. Those resources are also needed for other crucial social programs, like education, environmental protection, and so forth.

Because dollars are spent on unnecessary tests like the ones that saved my life, health insurance is expensive, and thousands of people can't afford to pay for it. And the costs of government health programs like Medicare and Medicaid are out of control because too much is spent on tests that have little or no medical justification. The fact that my life was saved by our system does not mean it was appropriate or defensible to do so. The end does not justify the means.

In my view, the CT scan that detected my kidney cancer was an abuse of the system. As a patient, I wasn't about to blow the whistle on the apparent abuse. But if I were acting as an attending physician and one of my residents told me that a patient was in the emergency room with his tenth kidney stone, and said, "we're getting a CT scan," I would respond with a stern and lengthy lecture on why that was a problematic decision.

All I can say to defend myself is that I actively opposed the unnecessary testing I received. If my insurance company had refused to pay for the tests, I would have accepted that decision without argument. If the company had required me to pay a big portion of the costs, I would have declined the tests. I do not think I was entitled to such services. Instead, I think they are good examples (although not the most dramatic ones) of what is happening in our out-of-control health care system.

At a medical ethics conference, I once heard the eminent economist Lester Thurow make similar points about his wife's kidney dialysis. He was speaking in the early 1970s, just after Congress voted to cover dialysis costs for any patient who needed this relatively expensive procedure. He said that he and his wife were very glad that she was able to obtain this lifesaving treatment. Nevertheless, he thought it was wrong for the government to use tax dollars to pay for every patient's dialysis when limited resources were needed to cover more urgent and justifiable social needs. The resources going to help his wife would be better spent on other things, he said.

LATE (AND LESS LUCKY) DIAGNOSIS

Two others in our group, Arthur Frank and Rebecca Dresser, followed longer and harder paths to diagnosis than I did. I had the personal good fortune to have an arguably unnecessary scan that revealed cancer, but they weren't as lucky as I was. While my cancer was diagnosed earlier than it really should have been, theirs was diagnosed after months of seeing doctors about disturbing symptoms. The tests and examinations needed to diagnose their cancer came late in the process.

Art's diagnosis began when he noticed soreness and what felt like a ridge in one of his testicles. In a state of anxiety, he visited his family doctor. The doctor thought it might be *Chlamydia*, an infectious disease easily treated with medication. But medication didn't do any good, and Art's condition became quite painful. Because Art was an athlete training for a triathlon, his doctor suggested the problem could be sports-related. He sent Art to a sports medicine specialist, who did a thorough physical examination and concluded that cancer was a possibility. That doctor ordered an ultrasound, which revealed abdominal tumors.

Now, it was clear that Art had cancer, but it wasn't clear what kind of cancer he had. By this time, he was in the hospital. His pain was excruciating, but the doctors still couldn't figure out exactly what was going on. When a surgeon recommended exploratory abdominal surgery to locate the primary tumor, Art refused to sign the consent form. He didn't think any of the several doctors he had seen had done the careful examination necessary to detect testicular cancer. And he was right. When a urologist was finally called in to examine him, that doctor made a quick (and correct) diagnosis of testicular cancer.[1]

Rebecca had a somewhat similar diagnostic odyssey. Hers began when she noticed ear pain and a strange feeling in her tongue. Her primary care doctor couldn't find anything wrong and suggested a visit to an ear, nose, and throat specialist. But the specialist, whose main clientele seemed to be children with earaches, didn't detect any problems. He said that if she was really worried about her symptoms, he could arrange for her to have a CT scan. But it was clear to Rebecca that he thought a scan was unnecessary. She hesitated to question his professional judgment, and didn't want him to think she was a hypochondriac. She was also relieved that he hadn't found anything serious—he had said what she wanted to hear. And like me, she was concerned about the proliferation of unnecessary and expensive testing that goes on in this country. So, she didn't push him to order the scan.

The specialist sent her away, without encouraging her to return if her symptoms got worse. They did get worse, but she wasn't sure what to do. She asked her dentist about them, but that didn't help, either. Her diagnosis was delayed for several months until she went back to her primary care doctor. At that point, she was sent to a distinguished specialist, who recognized her cancer almost immediately.

I had a similar experience regarding my rising platelet counts. Plenty of physicians looked at my CBC test results. Any one of them could have, and arguably should have, noticed that my platelet count was well above normal and getting higher all the time. Yet no doctor ever mentioned this to me. I don't know whether they missed it altogether, or whether they noticed it but kept silent. It's possible that they thought I would deal with it myself, since I was a doctor. And, eventually, I did deal with it. I referred myself to the blood specialist, who saw the danger and eventually prescribed the appropriate treatment. But I wonder what would have happened had I not been a physician, more curious and more knowledgeable about my test results than are most patients.

Their experiences with cancer diagnosis left Art and Rebecca feeling betrayed. They had expected doctors to diagnose their conditions promptly and accurately, but later realized this was a naïve expectation. Now they know that several things can get in the way of a prompt and accurate diagnosis. Doctors look for common conditions before considering more unusual ones—medical students and residents are repeatedly told, "when you hear hoof-beats, think about horses, not zebras."[2] Not all doctors examine patients as closely as they should, and some send patients away without advising them to return if symptoms don't improve. Once one doctor rules out a diagnosis, others tend to rely on that sometimes mistaken judgment. And even competent doctors can miss a diagnosis. In reality, patients are in the hands of a frighteningly imperfect medical system.[3]

Late (and perhaps mismanaged) diagnoses are difficult for patients. Besides having to cope with the burdens of advanced cancer, patients must cope with emotional fallout from the experience. They wonder whether they were given substandard care by doctors who didn't take their symptoms seriously. Relatively few patients are able to find out whether this happened, however. For example, Rebecca asked the doctor who diagnosed her cancer whether it should have been discovered sooner, but he couldn't give her a clear answer. He said that he couldn't be sure, because tumors like hers could be hard to detect.

In our litigious society, patients who suspect doctors of substandard practice sometimes sue those doctors. At one of our group meetings, I asked Art and Rebecca whether they had thought about bringing a lawsuit. Neither of them had considered taking legal action. Above all, they wanted to get through treatment and back to ordinary life. Achieving those goals took all of their available time and energy. Rebecca contemplated writing an angry letter to the specialist who had dismissed her concerns, but she was exhausted by treatment demands and wasn't sure whether he was at fault for missing the diagnosis. So, she tried to put aside her anger and concentrate on her recovery.

Their slow paths to diagnosis left Art and Rebecca painfully aware of their vulnerability as patients. Indeed, everyone in our group said their cancer experiences brought home how utterly dependent patients are on doctors and nurses. Even a patient like me, a person with extensive medical training and experience, must at some point put himself in the hands of his doctors and trust that they know what they're doing. And, fortunately, most of the time, they do. Sometimes they do not, however, and that's when people help themselves by becoming difficult patients. For example, it was Art's refusal to sign the surgical consent form that convinced doctors to call in a colleague who could make the right diagnosis. Art knew that a part of his body didn't feel right and by being stubborn, he compelled the doctors to pay attention to his belief. Rebecca sensed that something was wrong with her, too, but failed to challenge the doctor who dismissed her concerns.

Rebecca was not unusual in failing to challenge her doctor. I have seen many otherwise assertive and confident people become passive and child-like when they are dealing with doctors, and I have done this myself. Although doctors may have lost some of their former mystique, plenty of it remains. Among patients, there is an almost universal desire to be a good patient, someone the doctors will care enough about to put forth their best efforts. Doctors have charge of what matters most—a person's life and health. There is an understandable reluctance to question a doctor's judgment when doing so could threaten the relationship.

Patients have other reasons to defer to doctors who downplay their symptoms. Rebecca's failure to question her doctor was partly the result of her own wish to be told that she was okay. In his book, *At the Will of the Body*, Art wrote of his relief at hearing his initial diagnosis of *Chlamydia*, and of clinging to that diagnosis for a couple of weeks because it meant he didn't have cancer. In the next chapter, "Learning the Bad News," John Robertson writes of the role denial played in his failure to ask his wife, Carlota Smith, about the changes in her appearance that signaled cancer.

Physicians are susceptible to denying their symptoms, too. Doctors tend to consider themselves invincible, despite overwhelming evidence to the contrary. I have seen many members of the medical profession act as though they were immune to the illnesses that plague every other person on the planet. In his chapter, John tells the story of a famous cancer expert who put off seeing a doctor about his own cancer symptoms, symptoms that were obvious enough to alarm his family and colleagues. And I know from personal experience that medical training doesn't keep doctors from engaging in denial. For several months, I ignored the two mini-strokes I referred to earlier. Although I knew I had experienced all of the classic symptoms of a mini-stroke, I told myself that my symptoms were probably related to the occasional migraine attacks I have had throughout my life. For many months,

I also dismissed the rising platelet counts in my CBC reports as possible laboratory errors, or as part of the normal distribution curve.

It's common for patients and family members to blame themselves for contributing to a delayed diagnosis. Although this is understandable, I don't think they should be so hard on themselves. Our fears about cancer and other potentially deadly diseases are powerful, and they are widespread. They are powerful enough to drive the behavior of even doctors like me, who ought to know better. It's good to educate people about the warning signs of cancer, and to encourage them to seek medical attention when they notice one of them. But education won't always succeed in countering the strong psychological forces that can make people reluctant to respond to cancer symptoms.

THE PERILS OF EARLY DIAGNOSIS

Late diagnosis imposes heavy burdens on patients, but early diagnosis can be bad for patients, too. Two members of our group had their cancer diagnosed as a result of screening tests. In his chapter, "Coping with Uncertainty," Dan Brock describes how the results of a prostate specific antigen (PSA) test led to his prostate cancer diagnosis. Patricia Marshall's breast cancer was diagnosed after her annual mammogram revealed a possible tumor. In each case, screening did what it is supposed to do: detect cancer at a treatable stage. Both were treated for their cancer, and so far, treatment has been effective.

In one sense, Dan and Patty are "poster children" for cancer screening. In their cases, screening detected cancer, and the cancer was treated successfully. But an early diagnosis like Dan's isn't necessarily cause for celebration. On the one hand, Dan might not be alive today if he hadn't had the PSA test that led to the diagnosis. On other hand, he might be alive and well, without the disabling side effects that resulted from his surgery.

We know that much of the prostate cancer detected through PSA screening is not actually life-threatening. As Dan observes, men are more likely to die with prostate cancer than from it. Dan might have been better off without the test, although there is no way to know for sure. As long as doctors are uncertain which prostate cancers are aggressive and which are not, early prostate cancer diagnosis will lead to unnecessary and disabling treatment for thousands of men.

Similarly, screening mammography doesn't always benefit women. It misses some cancers (false-negative results) and identifies some "cancers" that really aren't there (false-positive results). False-positive results generate much anxiety, but can usually be corrected through further testing. The biggest problem with screening mammography is that it leads to overtreatment of some women who do have cancer. Some women undergoing burdensome and costly cancer treatment have tumors that would never become life-threatening. The exact size of this group is unknown, but it could be a substantial portion of the women who are treated.[4] But, as with prostate cancer, doctors often cannot tell which breast tumors can be left alone and which will become life-threatening without treatment. As a result, many women go through burdensome and risky cancer treatment that they don't really need.

The early diagnosis that prostate and breast cancer screening makes possible is a mixed blessing for patients and society. Early diagnosis saves some patients' lives, but this benefit comes at a price. Men and women who are treated unnecessarily pay a high personal price for that benefit, and the health care system pays a high monetary price for it.

THE MESSY REALITY OF DIAGNOSIS

Our group's experiences mark important realities about cancer diagnosis. One is that seeing a doctor doesn't necessarily lead to prompt and accurate diagnosis. When diagnosis is delayed, patients lose trust in the medical system. There is some benefit in this, for patients should sometimes be skeptical of the medical advice they receive. But patients have a hard time knowing when to be skeptical. Even privileged and educated patients are extremely dependent on the skills and attentiveness of the clinicians charged with their care. And even privileged and educated patients are susceptible to the denial that can contribute to a late cancer diagnosis.

At the other end of the spectrum is early cancer diagnosis. Early diagnosis can be a blessing, as it was for me. I probably wouldn't be alive if my kidney cancer had been diagnosed later than it was. But diagnoses like mine come at a price that our society cannot afford. It's unfair that I received the sort of unwarranted, unjustified test that is bankrupting our health care system. Early diagnosis isn't always good for patients, either. Some patients who are diagnosed early end up having harmful treatments they actually don't need.

As our group learned, diagnosis often depends on fortuities, like whether you happen to see a mediocre or a first-class physician, or whether the physician you see is conservative or liberal about ordering the expensive tests that can indicate cancer. Diagnosis also depends on a nation's value choices, such as whether it is more important to provide lavish care to people fortunate enough to have health coverage than to provide less-expensive but reasonable care to everyone. In my opinion, our current system is based on the wrong value choice. Today, too many people lack the health coverage that promotes appropriate cancer diagnosis, while privileged people like me get expensive and medically unnecessary tests that every once in a while reveal cancer.

Notes

1. Art describes his diagnosis in more detail in *At the Will of the Body* (New York: Houghton Mifflin, 1991, 2nd ed., 2002), 22–28.
2. See Jerome Groopman, *How Doctors Think* (New York: Houghton Mifflin, 2007), 126–127.
3. Many of these problems are described in Groopman, *How Doctors Think*.
4. See Steven Woloshin and Lisa Schwartz, "The Benefits and Harms of Mammography Screening," *JAMA* 303 (2010): 164–165.

CHAPTER 3

Learning the Bad News

John A. Robertson

It was May 23, 2010, three years after my wife, Carlota Smith, died of ovarian cancer. I was at home in Austin, Texas, reading my local Sunday paper and there it was: the death notice for Cheri Lin DeGreve, age forty-seven, who "died on Wednesday, May 12, 2010, following a three-year battle with ovarian cancer." Cheri was survived by her husband and two sons, parents, siblings, extended family, and many friends. A computer programmer, she had spent "the last thirteen years being the world's greatest stay-at-home mother and wife." The notice thanked a physician and nurse for "their professional and compassionate care." Cheri had "viewed [them] as her personal angels on earth."[1]

I felt great sadness for the DeGreve family. I wanted to tell them that I knew the pain and sadness they were experiencing and the world of grief they had just entered. The next day would be the third anniversary of Carlota's death. I had been there. I had experienced, as they had, the sudden, unexpected diagnosis, the poor prognosis, and the battles and heartache beyond. Cheri, like Carlota, was among the 21,500 women diagnosed with ovarian cancer and the 14,600 who die from this silent killer each year, a disease that strikes without warning and is fatal in 80% of the cases within five years.[2]

Cheri DeGreve had done better than Carlota and I had—Cheri had lived for three years after her diagnosis, while Carlota had lived for only two. But Carlota was seventy-three when she died, not forty-seven. She had twenty-six more years of life, enough to see her children grow up and have their own children and enough to have the rich professional career she kept up until three days before she died.

I have no idea how Cheri DeGreve discovered her cancer, but I suspect there is a compelling story about her diagnosis. Every patient and family has a story of how the cancer came to be identified and how they responded to the diagnosis. For Carlota and me, and Carlota's children and friends, it was unique and special, as if no one had ever experienced what we went through. Yet, millions had done so before us, as will millions in the future.

There are many different paths to the cancer diagnosis. A lump, a bump, a recurring redness, a sharp pain, a fever, a swelling, a cough, a shadow on an x-ray. In the previous chapter, "Diagnostic Quests and Accidents," Norman Fost describes his experience as one of the lucky patients whose early-stage cancer is discovered in the course of an unrelated test or examination. Carlota and I, as well as some of the others in our cancer ethics group, were not so lucky.

For the unlucky patients, the diagnosis comes later, often after symptoms were ignored or neglected for months. In our case, the news of cancer was the beginning of a personal tragedy: We were sucked into the fray, into the maelstrom from which we never fully escaped. When the diagnosis comes late, there can be guilt about not recognizing symptoms earlier and not pushing a loved one to see a doctor. This was my experience. I felt that since I was a medical ethicist who worked at the borders of health and illness, I should have known more, and pushed more, than I did.

Like 9/11 or President Kennedy's assassination, every cancer patient remembers the day and hour of the diagnosis. There are a thousand stories here. Although the stories have much in common, each is also unique. Each patient brings a different history, character, and set of relationships to the cancer diagnosis. Ovarian cancer has its own way of pulling patients into the swirling eddy, and other cancers have their ways. In the pages that follow, I tell my own story, my own variation on the sad tale of discovering a "bad" cancer (yes, from my vantage point, there are "good" cancers), hard to treat and invincible.

THE DESCENT INTO CANCER

For Carlota and me, the descent began in May, 2005. Carlota, a linguistics professor at the University of Texas, and I had planned a trip to London that month. I was to speak at a conference and Carlota was coming along to celebrate her seventy-first birthday and partake of the theater and art she loved. The day before we were scheduled to leave, she told me that she hadn't been feeling well. Her stomach was swollen, and she had gone to see a family practitioner she had consulted before about colds and the like. The doctor had ordered an ultrasound and gotten the results, but told her it would be okay to go ahead with the trip. She could have more tests when she got back.

This news was a shock to me. I had noticed that Carlota's abdominal area was getting bigger, but she had a fine figure, and I was hesitant to comment on her weight. In the interests of marital harmony, I chose not to say anything. Carlota, a self-described "rhinoceros" who rarely complained about her aches and pains, hadn't been feeling well for a few months. A few weeks earlier, she had become sick while attending an out-of-town conference. She spent a day in bed, but then went on to Boston to visit her daughter Alison and her family. She hadn't felt well there either, but seemed to have recovered by the time she got home. Later, I learned that Alison had noticed Carlota's distended stomach and made Carlota promise to see a doctor when she returned to Austin.

I didn't know what to do. I was worried, but the London travel arrangements were set and Carlota insisted that we go. Carlota, famous in the family for having what we jokingly called a "whim of iron," was not going to back down. I did not have enough medical information to make a case for staying home. There was no one I could call and consult, and no time to come up with a persuasive reason to cancel the trip. In retrospect, I can see that neither Carlota nor I wanted to admit that something could be seriously wrong. So, pretending that everything would be fine, we went to London.

We saw some interesting art and a great performance of "Hedda Gabler" on Carlota's birthday. We enjoyed ourselves, but couldn't escape our anxiety. Carlota was becoming weaker each day, although she was still walking about and putting up a stalwart front. By the third day, it was obvious to me that things were not going well, that we should cut the trip short and come home early. We called from London on Saturday morning to schedule a computed tomography (CT) scan for Monday, the day after we would arrive home. But because we didn't receive a telephone message about scan preparations, the scan had to be postponed until the next day. This was one of many maddening delays we encountered in the days before and after Carlota's diagnosis.

After the scan, we met with Carlota's family practice doctor to discuss the results. He said that he didn't have the full scan report and that more tests would be needed to determine what was going on.

He advised us to see a specialist, although he wasn't sure whether the problem was gastrointestinal or gynecological. He arranged for an appointment with Carlota's gynecologist the next afternoon.

I know now that the family practitioner actually had the full report when we saw him. He knew that Carlota had advanced cancer. But he couldn't bear to tell us the bad news. Later, after I discovered that he had had the report, I was furious at him for not being more forthcoming. I was also angry that he had concealed the ultrasound results and told Carlota to go ahead with the London trip. His evasive behavior delayed the scan and diagnosis for more than a week. I am a little less angry now, for I can see that it was probably beyond his expertise to tell his patient about a massive and serious cancer. A family practitioner would be unable to explain the condition and its treatment as well as a specialist could. And I know now that having the scan a week sooner would not have made much difference. At one level, I can excuse his behavior. Yet, I still think he did a poor job fulfilling his responsibilities as Carlota's primary care physician. As I discuss later, a good doctor would have handled the situation with more honesty and sensitivity than he did.

The next afternoon, we saw Carlota's gynecologist, who did not mince words. Directly and forcefully, she announced that Carlota's abdomen was full of cancer. I couldn't believe what I was hearing. In the uneasy days before the diagnosis, we had begun to suspect that Carlota might be seriously ill, but I had not thought specifically of cancer. The gynecologist recommended that we see a local specialist in gynecological cancer as soon as possible.

Left alone in the office for a minute, I went to hug Carlota, but she brushed me aside. She couldn't deal with the enormity of what we had just heard and wanted to escape to the outside world. And her gynecologist did nothing to cushion the blow. She offered no words of support, just made the appointment with the specialist and got us out of there. The specialist couldn't see us right away, so we had to suffer through a few more days of anxiety and uncertainty about how serious Carlota's condition really was.

When we finally made it to the appointment late on the Friday before Memorial Day weekend, the gynecological oncologist was forthright. After examining Carlota, looking at the scan, and reading the radiology report, she said there was tumor all over Carlota's abdomen, including the omentum (a term that refers to part of the peritoneum, one I had never heard in my thirty years in bioethics). The cancer appeared quite advanced and what to do about it was unclear.

Ordinarily, the doctor would perform surgery, but Carlota's abdomen was so full of fluid that an operation would be long, difficult, and risky. One alternative was to try chemotherapy first, which might reduce the fluid and make surgery more manageable.

Since we weren't far away from M. D. Anderson, the renowned cancer center in Houston, I asked the doctor what she thought they would say there. "Let's find out," she replied. She picked up the telephone and called the gynecological oncology department there. On the afternoon before the long holiday weekend, it took a while to locate a qualified doctor. But she finally reached an appropriate consultant and talked with him as we sat and waited. The expert thought it was reasonable to try chemotherapy as a way of making the surgery easier to do. But he also said there was no evidence that this approach would lengthen the patient's survival.

After a few minutes, with little discussion, we agreed to try chemotherapy first. The situation seemed urgent, and I assumed that we would start treatment the next day. But the oncologist said that because the cancer center was closed for Memorial Day, we would have to wait until Tuesday morning to begin. I was upset about the delay. The doctor explained that she could arrange for immediate chemotherapy at a local hospital, but Carlota would receive higher-quality care at the cancer center, a place that specialized in cancer treatment. So, we agreed to wait until Tuesday. The one positive development was that doctor was able to make Carlota more comfortable by draining some of the abundant fluid in her stomach.

We had the long Memorial Day weekend to endure before starting a possibly fruitless course of chemotherapy. To make things worse, we had scheduled a dinner party for Sunday night. I urged Carlota to cancel the party, but she refused. We ended up ordering pizza and making salad, telling people that something had come up that prevented us from cooking. One guest suspected that something was afoot and asked me about it, but Carlota and I had agreed to keep the diagnosis to ourselves. We both needed time to absorb what was happening and figure out how we should go about making our private nightmare public.

On Tuesday morning, we drove to the cancer center for what would be the first of many courses of chemotherapy we would have there. While we waited to get started, I went to the cancer center's social worker and told her how angry I was about all the delays we had encountered. Her only response was to give me information about a support group.

Once Carlota's treatment was under way, we received more signals that her condition was grave. One came from the gynecological oncologist who was now in charge of Carlota's treatment. As Carlota settled in to receive her first round of drugs, the oncologist came in and sat with us for a few minutes. I now realize that this was highly unusual. I never saw her in the chemotherapy suites again with any patient.

The conversation quickly turned to death. Carlota's doctor remarked that although many people think a sudden death is a good death, she thought that having time to say good-bye and settle accounts was in many ways better. As I tried to prolong the conversation and get details of what would happen next, it became clear that she wanted to leave (of course, she had other patients to see and there really was not much else to say). The message was clear, however. The doctor was preparing us for bad news and low expectations. But we did not grasp—or perhaps did not want to grasp—the full implications.

We received another signal that evening. Carlota developed a 104-degree fever in reaction to the chemotherapy drugs. We had been told to call the oncologist if this occurred. It took a while to reach the doctor, the first of many such frustrations we experienced during Carlota's treatment. Once I spoke to the doctor, she told us to go to the emergency room immediately. There, in the course of examining Carlota, an emergency room physician said to her, "You have terminal cancer." This was a shock to us, because we hadn't yet thought of it that way. But this was apparently the diagnosis that Carlota's oncologist had relayed to her emergency room colleague. The brutality of his statement instilled in us a loathing of the emergency room, and we never went there again.

Later, we did get a little good news. Two cycles of chemotherapy succeeded in reducing the fluid enough to allow doctors to perform surgery. Carlota's cancer was so advanced that there was no possibility of "getting it all," which is what patients and families usually hope for from cancer surgery. Because there were so many tumors scattered throughout Carlota's abdomen, surgery could at best reduce their size and make them more susceptible to chemotherapy.

Tissue from the operation showed that Carlota had stage-four ovarian and peritoneal cancer, two serious and incurable diseases. Carlota's oncologist gave us the general statistics on survival but refused to make any predictions about Carlota's future. When I pressed her to sit down with me for a few minutes to discuss the case, she did say that she did not expect Carlota to "die in the next six months" and that she would get her back teaching again. This calmed me down a little, for I had begun to wonder whether I would lose Carlota even sooner than that.

BAD NEWS FROM THE PATIENT'S PERSPECTIVE

We know that we are mortal creatures, but most of the time we put this knowledge aside. Even though we should be prepared for it, the news of a serious cancer is earth-shattering. Patients and their families never forget the early days of diagnosis. And they never forget how their doctors conveyed the horrible message. But, as several people in our cancer and ethics group discovered, not every doctor appreciates the significance of the occasion.

All doctors want to heal their patients, but in many cases this is impossible. Nearly every doctor who sees patients for a living has to tell some of them that they have a life-threatening illness. Breaking bad news is one of the doctor's patient care responsibilities. But, as the members of our group can confirm, not every doctor knows how to do this very well.

Looking back, we see several different problems with the cancer news we were given. Some doctors failed to give us adequate information. They told us we had cancer, but failed to say what could be done about it. For example, a specialist reviewing his scan told Arthur Frank that he had cancer, but refused to say anything more. Art would have to wait to see a different doctor to learn more about the terrifying news he had just heard. In a similar vein, a doctor told Rebecca Dresser he was "pretty sure" she had cancer, but said nothing about what could be done if she did. She spent several days not knowing whether her disease was treatable or terminal. Art and Rebecca felt lost and abandoned after these incidents. Thinking back on his experience, Art remarked, "Bartenders are liable for their customers who drink too much and drive. What about physicians, who tell people they have cancer, and then just leave them to drive home?"[3]

Doctors harm patients when they deliver a cancer diagnosis without discussing treatment possibilities. When this happens, patients whose cancer can be treated suffer days of needless terror before learning their true prospects. When nothing is said about the future, patients with untreatable cancer suffer needlessly, too. At the very least, doctors can reassure patients that they will do everything they can to keep patients active and comfortable in whatever time remains. And, when doctors have reason to suspect cancer, but need more time to make a definitive diagnosis, they can still reassure patients. One of Art's doctors did exactly that after Art asked whether he might have cancer. The doctor responded, "Yes, it could be, but if it is, we'll be right there with you." More than two decades later, Art still remembers how much comfort he took from that statement.

Besides information, patients need support from doctors delivering bad news. Some members of our group had doctors who displayed surprising insensitivity. The gynecologist who told us that Carlota had cancer never said a word about how sorry she was to have to give us such devastating news. The emergency room doctor was even worse, with his terse statement that Carlota's condition was terminal. The doctor who discovered Norm Fost's cancer had a technician call to tell Norm there was "something unusual" about his scan. Knowing how unsettling the message would be for a patient, a doctor with empathy would have made the call himself. A doctor who did take the trouble to call Patricia Marshall about her diagnosis brushed off Patty's nervous questions, cheerfully insisting there was nothing to worry about—again, a startling lack of empathy for a patient who had just learned she had breast cancer. These doctors were woefully out of touch with their patients.

Then there was the evasive behavior of Carlota's family practice doctor. This was the worst of the behavior that Carlota and I encountered. Doctors who dodge their responsibility to deliver bad news harm not only their patients, but their colleagues, too. Danielle Ofri, a physician at New York University, writes of her rage at having to stand in for doctors in another part of the hospital who failed to tell a patient, Ramonita Ortega, that her X-ray revealed lung cancer. "How," she asked, "could they have done this to Ms. Ortega? And how could they have put me in this position . . .?"[4] The doctors who read the X-ray "made the proper referral to an internist, but slunk away from the messier part," the part that required them to talk to their patient. Seething at their moral cowardice, Ofri delivered the bad news as best she could.

As bad as they were, our experiences with cancer diagnosis could have been worse. After Carlota's death, a friend came to me with his own diagnosis story. An oncologist was delivering bad news to my friend and his wife, the parents of two children in grade school. The doctor said that my friend's wife had serious abdominal cancer. To convey the gravity of the situation, he said, "There is a 50% chance that you won't live to see your daughter graduate from high school." That cut my friend and his wife to the quick. My friend was still angry and the tears flowed as he relayed those words to me a week later. What insensitivity to put the facts in that most brutal way, when there were gentler ways to put it! Surely oncologists are taught how to talk to patients better than that.

WHAT DOCTORS SHOULD KNOW

Unfortunately, many patients can tell stories about the insensitive and maladroit behavior exhibited by the doctors who told them they had cancer. It's not clear that individual doctors, or the profession as a whole, give breaking bad news the priority it deserves. We believe that the doctor's skill in delivering bad news is as important as any of the skills involved in the happier sides of medical practice. Yet, our own experiences and others we have heard and read about are evidence that too many doctors do a poor job breaking bad news.

Since delivering bad news is something that oncologists do often, they should do it well. But it is a complex process, laden with emotion and the potential for misunderstanding. With the exception of a few gifted men and women who perform well on their own, doctors need instruction in handling this difficult task.

To its credit, the medical profession now recognizes that doctors need to get better at delivering bad news. Researchers have begun to collect data designed to help with this process. Studies show that patients diagnosed with cancer want prompt and comprehensive information about their condition and prognosis. They want their doctors to help them understand the medical facts, and they want help in thinking through or coming to terms with what will happen next. Patients say they do best when they receive technical information that helps them plan and deal with the future. In fact, in one study patients rated information about their disease and its treatment as more important than support from the physician. Patients still ranked support as important or very important, though, indicating that they want both facts and empathy from their doctors.[5]

Using information like this, clinicians have developed tools designed to improve the way doctors deliver bad news like a cancer diagnosis. An approach called SPIKES divides breaking bad news into six steps: (1) setting up the interview; (2) assessing patients' perceptions of their medical situations; (3) inviting patients to indicate how much information they would like; (4) giving patients knowledge about their disease; (5) addressing patients' emotions; and (6) summarizing a strategy for the future. The approach offers guidelines for each step. For example, in setting up the interview, the doctor should find a private setting, sit down with the patient, maintain eye contact, and minimize interruptions.[6]

Creators of the SPIKES protocol see step five, addressing the patient's emotions, as one of the most difficult parts of delivering a cancer diagnosis. Patients respond to the diagnosis in different ways. Some shut down, some express great sadness or anger, and some can't believe what they have just heard. The SPIKES guidelines advise doctors to pay close attention to the individual patient, talking with her about how she feels and why she is feeling that way. In the words of the clinicians who developed SPIKES:

> Patients regard their oncologist as one of their most important sources of psychological support, and combining empathic, exploratory, and validating statements is one of the most powerful ways of providing that support. It reduces the patient's isolation, expresses solidarity, and validates the patient's feelings or thoughts as normal or to be expected.[7]

The emergence of guidelines like these makes it possible for physicians to become better at breaking bad news. Although there are limits to any "cookbook" approach, doctors following the SPIKES guidelines will be better at delivering a cancer diagnosis than were several of the doctors our group members encountered. Every doctor involved in patient care should take the time to learn these techniques. In my view, training for oncologists ought to be mandatory, since so much of their job involves delivering bad news. Besides disclosing the initial diagnosis, oncologists must deliver bad news to patients later on, when cancer comes back or spreads, treatment fails, treatment side effects are irreversible, or all treatment options have been exhausted.[8]

BAD NEWS AND HOPE

A cancer diagnosis is never good news, but there are many kinds and stages of cancer. My previous points pertain to disclosures about cancer generally, affecting patients with any type and stage of cancer. What made the news so bad for Carlota and for me was the absence of any effective long-term treatment for her cancer. Although Carlota's cancer diagnosis could have been handled better, our suffering had to do less with how the grim diagnosis was communicated than with its grim content.

In communicating bad news, especially when the news is as grim as it was for Carlota and me, doctors must help people hold on to hope. The best way to do this, writes physician Chris Feudtner, is for doctors to respect "the breadth of hopes."[9] Doctors who ask patients and families what they hope for will find that "hope in the big sense is actually composed of multiple hopes in the smaller sense." When an illness is life-threatening and treatment options are limited, patients and families will often admit that they hope for a miracle. But, they will also have what Feudtner calls "smaller hopes," such as hope that the patient can be kept comfortable and hope for a few more months of survival.

Doctors can do a lot to make these smaller hopes a reality. And even hope for a miracle deserves the clinician's respect, for it can help people get through the ordeal of a serious illness. "Judging such a hope as either realistic or false misses the point," Feudtner contends. Instead, he writes, "we should judge ourselves as clinicians by the degree to which we can help nurture our patients' collections of diverse hopes."[10]

Feudtner is not the only clinician who thinks doctors should explicitly address hope when they talk with patients about a serious diagnosis. Some see this as an essential part of breaking bad news. Besides discussing diagnosis and prognosis, they say, breaking bad news requires "salvage—statements intended to reduce the impact of the bad news and help the patient and family cope with a life-altering diagnosis."[11] Engaging in salvage requires doctors to help patients and families transform their previous hopes for long life into hopes that are achievable in their new reality. Sustaining hope in these circumstances also demands sensitivity: "When the physician forms an empathic emotional connection with the patient, it conveys an unspoken but important message of caring: the physician's steady presence is an almost physical shelter in the emotional storm that often accompanies impending death."[12]

Carlota and I maintained hope throughout her illness, sometimes for realistic goals and sometimes for what we knew wasn't possible. None of our doctors asked Carlota and me to talk about our hopes, which points to a gap between the recommendations I just described and the reality that many patients experience. Yet, I can see now that Carlota's oncologist did try to focus our attention on smaller hopes, such as getting Carlota back to work. I also realize that her conversation with us that the first day of chemotherapy was meant to show us what we could reasonably hope for in our new circumstances.

She never took away our hope for more time, but she illuminated the other things we could hope for, like having time to say good-bye.

DIAGNOSIS AND DENIAL

For me, the worst parts of the diagnosis involved denial and delay. Carlota and I both denied her symptoms, and we paid for it. In the awful days after her diagnosis, I was angry with Carlota for not telling me about her symptoms sooner. I was also angry with myself. I felt tremendously guilty that I had not paid more attention to the signs and symptoms of Carlota's illness.

I felt that as a person with some knowledge of medical matters, I should have pushed through the denial and got her examined earlier. Although it might not have made much difference, it has taken me three years to get over my guilt for failing to intervene.

But I can see now that Carlota and I were not the only ones who had trouble facing her cancer. The family practitioner did not want to confront what he had uncovered; instead, he sought to pass the burden to someone else. Carlota's gynecologist did not try to duck her responsibility, but after she announced the bad news, she left the office, unwilling to stay with us as we absorbed her terrible words. In contrast, the gynecological oncologist did several things to show us she recognized the gravity of our situation. She was kind and empathic at our first appointment, taking the time to drain fluid so that Carlota would be more comfortable during the long weekend before we began chemotherapy. She also deserves praise for coming to the chemotherapy room to talk with us during that first session. It took courage for her to bring up the topic of dying so early in the relationship. This was, in my view, a caring way to help us face our new reality.

A biography I read after Carlota's death also helped me to understand that Carlota and I were far from alone in letting denial get in the way of a cancer diagnosis. Henry Kaplan was a well-known radiologist who made important advances in treating Hodgkin's disease in the 1960s and 1970s. Then he was diagnosed with lung cancer. As his biographer put it, "September 28, 1983, marked the time his life changed forever."[13]

Henry Kaplan was a professional trained to know the symptoms of cancer. But he refused to recognize those symptoms in himself. For several months, he ignored a raspy cough, as well as pleas from his wife and colleagues to see a doctor about it. When he finally decided to seek medical attention, he handled the diagnosis in a distinctively personal way. He had a chest X-ray and then read it himself. Although he saw a baseball-size tumor in his left lung, colleagues reported he showed no reaction. He simply moved on to the next step in his evaluation, calling a chest radiologist for a needle biopsy and arranging for a scan to see if the tumor had spread. A doctor present at the time reports a lasting image of Henry Kaplan with several other radiologists, "discussing his scans as though he were consulting on some other patient."[14] A surgeon involved in Kaplan's care remarked on how dispassionate he seemed: "He provided a complete history, as if talking about another patient. . . . He was going to make all the decisions and that was that."[15]

But even Henry Kaplan had his limits. He was able to maintain a detached perspective the next day when he called his laboratory staff together and told them about his diagnosis. Then his professional mask slipped:

> [W]hen [his daughter] Annie came in a few minutes later, he couldn't speak. He just put his arms around her. For the first time, his wife, Leah, openly sobbed. "It broke my heart," she said. Soon they were all crying. Henry had handled his diagnosis well as a physician, colleague, neighbor, and even husband. But as a father he could no longer suppress his grief.[16]

I found solace in this account because it showed me how widespread denial is and how many people have postponed their diagnosis and perhaps shortened their lives because they couldn't admit that they might be ill. Here was an internationally renowned oncologist who fought day and night to advance cancer treatment. Kaplan was totally committed to his patients, yet he failed to acknowledge his own symptoms. Earlier attention might have given him more months, just as it might have given Carlota and me more time. On the other hand, it might not have given any of us more time. Kaplan's story helped me put aside my desire to blame someone—myself, Carlota, a doctor—for what happened to Carlota and me.

Kaplan's story also helped me to see how a person's character and personality determine the way that person reacts to and copes with dire news. Carlota, like Henry Kaplan, took a detached professional stance. Indeed, she never broke down and sobbed with her children or with me. She kept on in her professional work. She always had hope, if only for a few months more of life. Even when she knew the beast was loose inside her and growing rapidly, she kept doing the things she loved.

CLOSING THOUGHTS

Three years after Carlota's death, I still have strong feelings about what we experienced as her disease entered our lives and a definite diagnosis emerged. At the time, I was tremendously angry at the family practitioner for saying we could go to London and for not being straight with us when we got back. I believe that he lied to us about what was in the report on that first CT scan. He must have recognized that it showed she had cancer. And did he really think it was okay for Carlota to go on the trip? Why didn't he call me in too, or tell her to see her gynecologist right away?

Now, however, I am able to be a bit more understanding about the family practitioner's behavior. Perhaps he was out of his depth. His family practice training probably had not prepared him to talk with patients with a disease as serious and complicated as Carlota's was. Moreover, he had only the scan report, and any meaningful discussion of her disease, prognosis, and treatment options would have to be led by the proper specialist. So, I did come to see how difficult it would have been for him to reveal Carlota's diagnosis. I also realize that getting the diagnosis a couple of weeks earlier would not have made much difference in the ultimate outcome.

Despite this, I wish that the doctor had been more caring and supportive. He just handed us off to the other doctors. And he never reached out again, although he had been Carlota's first-line doctor for several years. I am left with a feeling that he should have handled it better. As I should have handled it better. Just as I am weak and limited, he is as well. So, I accept and forgive.

At this point, I can also see that a doctor's honesty and compassion go only so far. When patients and their families hear the bad news about cancer, they will inevitably feel devastated. In that awful summer of 2005, after the diagnosis and during the chemotherapy that preceded Carlota's surgery, I found myself drawn to an incident in Herman Melville's novel, *Moby Dick*. The novel describes a longboat that has gone in pursuit of a whale and is caught in a squall at night. The boat is cut off from the mother ship and the other longboats, perhaps lost forever. Starbuck manages to light a candle and put it in a box on a pole. He gives the pole to Queequeg to hold up as a beacon in the darkness. In Melville's words, he "handed it to Queequeg as the standard bearer of this forlorn hope. There, then, he sat, the sign and symbol of a man without faith, hopelessly holding up hope in the midst of despair."[17]

To me, Queequeg's demeanor and desperation are like those of the patients and families confronted with the diagnosis of advanced cancer. All that Carlota and I could do when we heard the fatal words of a stage-four cancer diagnosis was to hold up a candle in the storm. We could hope for a little more time, and we could hope for courage as we faced what was coming. We could go on, as Carlota did, "hopelessly holding up hope in the midst of despair."

Disclosure protocols and training may help doctors soften the blow of a cancer diagnosis, and this is definitely worth doing. To be honest, though, doctors cannot rescue patients and their loved ones from this agonizing personal tragedy. In the end, getting through the catastrophe of an advanced cancer is something each patient and family must do for themselves. We are all in that boat together.

Notes

1. "Funerals and Memorials," *Austin American-Statesman*, May 23, 2010, B4.
2. Marilynn Marchionne, "Ovarian Cancer Screening Shows Promise in Study," August 17, 2010. Retrieved May 20, 2010, from http://www.newsvine.com/_news/2010/05/20/4318402-overain-screening-shows-promise-in-study
3. The quotation is from a "found poem" that is based on an interview with Art. See Loreen Herwaldt, *Patient Listening: A Doctor's Guide* (Iowa City: University of Iowa Press, 2008), 38.
4. Danielle Ofri, "They Sent Me Here," *New England Journal of Medicine* 352 (2005): 1746–48.
5. The same study found varying preferences among patients from different demographic groups. Researchers reported that

   > female patients place more importance on getting detailed information about their cancer and on having the physician provide them support when being told the news than do male patients. In addition, patients with more formal education tended to want more information from their physicians and also indicated that the context of how the news was told was more important than patients with less formal education.

   Patricia A. Parker, Walter F. Baile, Carl de Moor, et al., "Breaking Bad News About Cancer: Patients' Preferences for Communication," *Journal of Clinical Oncology* 19 (2001): 2049–56.
6. Walter F. Baile, Robert Buckman, Renato Lenzi, et al., "SPIKES—A Six-Step Protocol for Delivering Bad News: Application to the Patient with Cancer," *The Oncologist* 5 (2000): 302–11.
7. Baile, et al., "SPIKES," 307.
8. Baile, et al., "SPIKES," 302.
9. Chris Feudtner, "The Breadth of Hopes," *New England Journal of Medicine* 361 (2009): 2306–2307.

10. Feudtner, "Breadth of Hopes," 2307.

11. Simon N. Whitney, Laurence B. McCullough, Ernest Fruge, et al., "Beyond Breaking Bad News: The Roles of Hope and Hopefulness," *Cancer* 113 (2008): 442–45, 444.

12. Whitney et al., "Beyond Breaking Bad News," 445.

13. Charlotte DeCroes Jacobs, *Henry Kaplan and the Story of Hodgkin's Disease* (Stanford, California: Stanford University Press, 2010), 376.

14. Jacobs, *Henry Kaplan*, 377.

15. Jacobs, *Henry Kaplan*, 377.

16. Jacobs, *Henry Kaplan*, 378.

17. I give the full quote, which has summed up so much of my experience with Carlota's cancer:

> The wind increased to a howl; the waves dashed their bucklers together; the whole squall roared, forked, and crackled around us like a white fire upon the prairie, in which, unconsumed, we were burning; immortal in these jaws of death. In vain we hailed the other boats; as well roar to the live coals down the chimney of a flaming furnace as hail those boats in that storm. Meanwhile the driving scud, rack, and mist, grew darker with the shadows of the night; no sign of the ship could be seen. The rising sea forbad all attempts to bail out the boat. The oars were useless as propellers, performing now the office of life preservers. So, cutting the lashing of the waterproof match keg, after many failures, Starbuck contrived to light the lamp in the lantern; then stretching it on a waif pole, handed it to Queequeg as the standard bearer of this forlorn hope. There, then, he sat, holding up that imbecile candle in the heart of that almighty forlornness. There, then, he sat, the sign and symbol of a man without faith, hopelessly holding up hope in the midst of despair.

Herman Melville, *Moby-Dick; or the Whale* (Berkeley, California: University of California Press, 1981), 230.

CHAPTER 4

Coping with Uncertainty

Dan W. Brock

In May of 2001, I was in Oxford, England, interviewing for a new teaching position in bioethics. Soon after the interview, they offered me the job. A couple of days later, I returned to my home in Providence, Rhode Island, and learned that I had prostate cancer. Truly a good-news, bad-news week. As far as I know, I never experienced any serious ethical lapses in my care, nor did I face any deeply problematic ethical choices in the course of my treatment. But I did experience repeated and difficult uncertainties in deciding how to proceed, which was probably the hardest part of the whole business.

In this chapter, I describe the uncertainties I faced when I had cancer, as well as uncertainties I faced after being diagnosed with a second serious illness. Before I was diagnosed with these conditions, I knew something about uncertainty in medicine and the problems this creates for doctors and patients. But becoming seriously ill taught me much more about the personal difficulties and distress that uncertainty creates for patients coping with chronic and life-threatening conditions.

QUESTIONS ABOUT PROSTATE CANCER TREATMENT

Prostate cancer is a slow-growing cancer, common in elderly men (I was sixty-three when I was diagnosed). Doctors disagree about whether, when, and how to treat it. The prostate specific antigen (PSA) test that led to my diagnosis is itself controversial, for it is unclear how much the PSA test improves life expectancy. Indeed, the 2001 PSA test that led to my diagnosis was the first one for me. Before that, my doctor had recommended against doing it because of its questionable benefit.

The first test showed that my PSA was only moderately elevated, but it was significantly higher in a second test. The PSA test can produce fluctuating results for a number of reasons, including some that have no medical significance. Thus, the implications of my PSA test results were uncertain. Despite the uncertainty, the urologist I had been referred to recommended that I have a prostate biopsy. This involves sampling cells from about a dozen places in the prostate. The biopsy found a relatively low number of tumor cells, all confined to one area of the prostate. My Gleason score, a measure of the cancer's aggressiveness, was in the middle range.

"Watchful waiting" is one possible alternative for prostate cancer, especially in elderly men.[1] Experts say that more men die with prostate cancer than from it. My urologist advised against watchful waiting, because my relatively young age and lack of other health problems meant that prostate cancer had a real possibility of shortening my life. Quite apart from his judgment on this, I think I would have found it very difficult to "leave it there" and do nothing. This is a reaction that many men with prostate cancer have to the watchful waiting alternative. People diagnosed with any kind of cancer generally want to do something to get rid of it.

After rejecting watchful waiting, I still faced a choice among several alternative interventions. I could have a surgical procedure called *radical prostatectomy*, which removes the entire prostate. There were also two forms of radiation therapy available to me—directed-beam radiation and radioactive seeds implanted in the prostate.

The choice I faced was shot through with uncertainty. First, there was disagreement about which treatment produced the lowest five-year recurrence rate. (After five years, experts believed patients were relatively home free.) Since the two methods of radiation were new in comparison with the surgery, less information was available on their outcomes. My urologic surgeon, not surprisingly, favored the surgical alternative of radical prostatectomy. To his credit, though, he sent me to meet with a radiologist to explore the radiological alternatives. I was pleased that my doctor recognized his possible treatment bias and encouraged contact with other doctors who might have different opinions. In my case, however, meeting with the radiologist did little to resolve my uncertainty about which treatment to choose.

I also turned to the Internet for help. I hoped that reading some of the medical literature on my cancer and its treatment might point me toward one of the options. The information I found was helpful, but hardly decisive. Eventually, I concluded (with much uncertainty) that a majority of experts regarded radical prostatectomy as the "gold standard," the alternative that was most likely to eliminate the cancer. I think this was partly because doctors were less familiar with and had less research data about the two forms of radiation. In contrast, surgery had been studied and used for a long time.

Besides facing uncertainty about which treatment would give me the best chance to survive, I faced uncertainty about the risks and side effects of each treatment option. Surgery seemed to have a bit higher risk of incontinence and impotence, the two most serious and common side effects of prostate cancer treatment. Again, however, there were conflicting data about their incidence. Doctors assured me that these side effects were quite unlikely in the nerve-sparing surgery I would undergo. But I've since concluded that they are probably more common than my doctors suggested. It seems to me that many doctors understate the risks of these side effects. When I was doing my research, I found one renowned specialist who claimed that less than 10% of his patients experienced incontinence and impotence, but other reports I read estimated that these side effects occurred in roughly 25% of surgery patients. Besides the higher risk of side effects, surgery would expose me to the risks of general anesthesia. Surgery would be more physically intrusive, too, and it would involve a longer recovery time than radiation would.

As I recall, I was told that with any of the treatments, the risk of cancer recurrence was around 20%, although that depended on how much cancer was in the prostate, as well as whether the cancer had spread beyond the prostate capsule to the lymph nodes. If I had surgery and the cancer recurred, I could then have radiation treatment. The reverse was apparently not true—surgery was not an effective option for recurrence after radiation. This seemed to me to be a significant advantage of the surgery.

Because prostate cancer is relatively common, I was able to talk to several friends who had once faced the same choice I was facing. Yet, this didn't help much, because their individual treatment choices were all different. Since I had been teaching at Brown University Medical School for nearly two decades, I could also seek advice from physicians I knew personally. But again, this didn't help much, because they simply did not agree on the best treatment alternative, either in general or in my particular case. Having learned to be good nonpaternalistic doctors, none of the doctors I consulted was prepared to push for a particular alternative. Perhaps this was right on their part, since none of the options was clearly superior and the decision was highly personal. But their reluctance to make recommendations did not make the decision any easier.

After a few weeks of research and conversation, I needed to make my decision. I was preparing to leave Brown to spend a year working at the National Institutes of Health (NIH) in Washington, D.C., and I wanted to resolve the issue before moving. I decided to have the surgery my urologist favored, hoping that it would be effective and that I would be one of the patients who escaped its most serious side effects.

The surgery turned out to be tougher than I had anticipated. The recovery period was longer and more demanding than I had been led to expect. I was in the hospital longer than usual, had significant pain, and in general felt poorly. I then recuperated at home for a couple of weeks, much of the time in bed. Immediately after the surgery, I was given a Foley catheter with a bag for collecting urine that remained in place for about two weeks. Although the doctors assured me that any incontinence and impotence I experienced would probably be temporary, they would not say how long the conditions would last. Apparently, continence and sexual potency can return almost immediately after surgery, or as much as a year later. This uncertainty was at least as bad as the earlier uncertainty about which treatment to pursue.

In the weeks that followed, I continued to have problems with incontinence. Nevertheless, my urologist continued to express hope that I would recover. During the first few months at NIH, I remained completely incontinent and had to wear diaper-like pads that I had to change several times a day. Even with the pads, I felt uncomfortable much of the time. The problem was not going away, and about a year after the surgery, my urologist finally acknowledged that I was unlikely to recover from the incontinence.

Because I was working in Washington, I went to a new urologist to see if I could get help for the incontinence, which I found very difficult and unpleasant to deal with. I knew there were some ways to treat the condition, although none seemed all that promising. One silver lining appeared at this point. The new urologist suggested surgery to insert an artificial sphincter, which turned out to be quite successful. This device allows me to control urination by pressing a button. Although there is some leakage, especially when I sit in certain ways that put pressure on the sphincter, I found it an enormous improvement. And later I learned of another silver lining. Because of the surgery, my PSA was very low, "like a girl's," as one physician put it. And so far, there is no evidence that my cancer has returned.

UNCERTAINTY IN MEDICINE

Perhaps one of the most important lessons I've learned in nearly three decades of working in medical ethics is how much uncertainty there is in the practice of medicine. Jay Katz and other medical ethicists have described in detail the problems this creates for patients.[2] Before becoming seriously ill, most patients are unaware of the uncertainties they will face. This lack of awareness leads many patients to conclude that any bad outcome means someone must have done something wrong. Few members of the general public appreciate the uncertainty that doctors confront in medical practice.

Medical ethicists argue that doctors and patients should make treatment decisions together, for several reasons. Because there are many medically accepted alternative treatments for common conditions, the best choice for a particular patient often depends on that patient's personal situation and values. Often no single alternative is best for all patients. This was the situation I faced with my prostate cancer.

I did not find my physicians, the Internet, or my friends who had had prostate cancer very helpful in dealing with the uncertainty. I have no easy solutions to this problem, but I am certain that uncertainty was the hardest part of the ordeal. Unlike several other patients in our cancer ethics group, my cancer treatment was neither prolonged nor very burdensome, except for the long-term side effects. Once I had the artificial sphincter, there were no more significant decisions to make about my prostate cancer. Even before I reached the five-year cancer-free mark, I thought of my cancer as "cured." I rarely worry or even think about it. In my mind, we went in and dealt with it, and it is gone, except for the side effects of the treatment. I am one of few former patients in our group who feel confident that their cancer is gone.

I am also one of the two people in our group for whom cancer was not such a "big deal." The reasons I feel this way are that prostate cancer is more successfully treated, and its treatment less burdensome, than any of the other cancers and treatments people in our group experienced. My treatment choices may have involved more uncertainty than those of some of the others, but even with the long-lasting side effects, the whole cancer experience was less arduous for me than it was for the others in our group.

But my relatively relaxed response to cancer surely grows out of something that happened to me after I had cancer. Four years after being treated for cancer, I faced another medical problem that seemed even more serious than cancer. It was a problem that also presented more uncertainty than my cancer had presented.

In 2004, while I was in Washington, my internist was doing a general examination and noticed something odd about the reflexes in my foot. He sent me to a neurologist, who arranged for me to have a full neurological exam, including a scan of the brain and spinal cord. The evaluation was inconclusive, and the doctors couldn't tell me what was causing my symptoms.

After the exam, I left Washington for a new job at the Harvard Medical School. A few months later, I noticed that I was having a little trouble walking. I saw a neurologist in Boston, and he concluded that I had probably had a small stroke. The following summer, while walking on a beach with friends, I noticed that I kept stumbling. Walking in the sand was considerably more difficult than it had been the previous summer. I went to see the neurologist again, and he sent me for a neuromuscular workup. After that, I learned that I probably had multiple sclerosis (MS).

To my dismay, I discovered that there is even more medical uncertainty about MS than there is about prostate cancer. First, it can take many years for patients to be diagnosed. It had been two years from the time my Washington doctor first noticed symptoms to my diagnosis of MS. So, I went through a long period of uncertainty about what was going on. In contrast, my prostate cancer was diagnosed and treated in only a couple of months. And my own diagnostic delay was much shorter than what many MS patients experience. Unlike prostate cancer, there is no blood test or biopsy to indicate whether MS is present. Although magnetic resonance imaging (MRI) scans have made the MS diagnosis easier and faster, MS remains a diagnosis of exclusion. This means that doctors diagnose it only after they exclude several other conditions that have similar symptoms.

Most patients with MS have what is called *relapsing and remitting MS*, which typically includes periods of symptom relief and can be treated with several different drugs. I have a more unusual form of the disease called *primary progressive MS* (PPMS). As the name implies, it takes a steady progressive course. Moreover, there are no effective medications to treat it. All of the promising drugs that have been studied have turned out to have no beneficial effects in PPMS patients. Although I have tried three different drugs that doctors suggested might help with symptoms, I did so knowing that they were unlikely to work (and, as I expected, they did not help). The one certainty in PPMS is that there are no good treatments.

What is most uncertain is how I will fare in the future. What patients with a serious chronic progressive disease like mine most want to know is the prognosis, especially when there is no proven effective treatment. But patients with PPMS get almost no solid information about their prognosis. Individual patients with this condition have quite varied symptoms. Many of the common symptoms can occur in nearly unlimited combinations in any specific patient. New symptoms can develop at any point as the disease progresses. Doctors can give patients no indication of which symptoms will develop over time, except that the ones they already have are likely to get worse. Patients are simply told, "Every patient is different."

More importantly, PPMS patients get no information about how fast their disease is likely to progress, other than that it is likely to progress at about the same speed that it has in the past. Again, there is much variation in how quickly the disease moves, from almost no progression to a very rapid and severe decline. About five years ago, I pressed my neurologist to give me some idea about my likely rate of progression. With some reluctance, he answered, "You will likely be using a cane in four years, and if you are alive in twenty years, you are likely to be in a wheelchair."

I have been using a cane now for about three years, so the neurologist's prediction was overly optimistic. And I see now that my quest for information was misconceived. Although I urged my doctor to give me an estimate at the time, I now question whether physicians should make, or allow themselves to be pushed to make, predictions about conditions like mine, where there is so little basis for knowing what will happen to an individual patient.

Coping with MS and the uncertainty about its future impact has been much tougher for me than was coping with the uncertainty about prostate cancer. The uncertainty about cancer treatment alternatives and side effects was hard to take, but the uncertainty ended after a couple of years and I could be pretty sure of what the future looked like. But with MS, the future is highly uncertain and unpredictable. Planning is extremely difficult. I have come to understand that most of the necessary coping and adjustment cannot be done in advance. I simply have to accept and live with this uncertainty about my future health and disability, making changes in my life and circumstances when they become necessary.

Of course, many cancer patients face the same sorts of uncertainty that I face with MS. Indeed, some of the other patients in our cancer ethics group think there is a reasonable chance that their cancers will come back. Having cancer, as well as other illnesses, has forced us to recognize that doctors cannot tell us exactly what future is in store for us. We must accept and adjust to what comes, whether we like it or not.

SHARED DECISION-MAKING AND UNCERTAINTY

Although I had read, taught, and written about uncertainty in medical decision-making before I faced serious illness, I did not fully appreciate the problems uncertainty presents for patients. The uncertainties I have described have been the most difficult aspects of my illnesses. Are there ways that physicians can do a better job of helping patients deal with uncertainty? Here, a bit of historical perspective may be useful.

Until the 1960s, the relationship between doctors and patients was based on paternalism and professional authority. Paternalism was seen as the proper ethical approach for doctors, and most doctors practiced in accord with this ethical judgment. According to medical tradition, the physician was the one who made the treatment decisions. He—and at that time it was usually a "he"—had the knowledge, training, and experience to diagnose the patient's condition and determine what treatment offered the best chance for improving that condition. Because patients lacked this knowledge, training, and experience, they did not play an active role in decisions about their care. The patients' role was to follow the doctor's orders. The only information patients needed was how to comply with those orders.

For the paternalistic medical system to work, patients had to trust their doctors. Patients had to believe that doctors were experts who knew what was best. If doctors shared their uncertainty about a patient's diagnosis or about which treatment would be best, patients would stop trusting their doctors. Doctors were afraid that being open about uncertainty might make patients less willing to follow doctors' orders. As a result, it was common for doctors to conceal any uncertainties they had about their patients' care.

By the time I confronted prostate cancer and MS, this vision of the doctor–patient relationship had been rejected. During the 1960s and 1970s, the civil rights movement and Vietnam War protests led people

52   *Malignant*

to question the authority of government and other leaders. Eventually, they began to question the authority of doctors, too. At the same time, research was beginning to produce many new treatments for medical conditions, including alternative treatments for the same medical condition. Sometimes there was no medical consensus about which alternative was best for all patients with a specific disease. For example, before the 1970s, most doctors thought that radical mastectomy was the best treatment for all women with breast cancer. But then new research showed that mastectomy and the less disfiguring alternative of lumpectomy produced about the same survival results. Similarly, by the time I was diagnosed with prostate cancer, several treatment alternatives seemed to produce about the same survival rates.

When no single treatment produces superior medical results, the choice among alternatives depends on the specific concerns and values of the individual patient. With breast cancer, for example, some women care more about preserving their breasts than others do. In the new era, patients have to be more involved in treatment decision-making because they, not their physicians, know which treatment best suits their individual situations.[3]

As a result of these developments, shared decision-making has replaced the paternalist, authoritarian model of the doctor–patient relationship.[4] In its simplest version, shared decision-making recognizes that both doctors and patients bring something distinct to treatment decision-making, that both have knowledge that is required for good treatment choices. Physicians bring their knowledge, training, and experience with the patient's medical condition and its treatment; this is why patients go to physicians. Patients bring knowledge of their specific values and concerns, knowledge that affects how they evaluate the risks and potential benefits of different treatment alternatives.

In the new model of shared decision-making, there is more openness about medical uncertainty. Yet, as Rebecca Dresser emphasizes in the next chapter, this doesn't mean that doctors must refrain from expressing an opinion on the best option for a patient. In the new model, physicians should feel free to make treatment recommendations (indeed, that is what patients seek from physicians) and should, in some circumstances, try to persuade patients to accept their recommendations. In turn, patients should feel free to rely on their physicians' recommendations. But, as the term implies, shared decision-making requires doctors to share medical knowledge with patients, and that includes revealing uncertainties and gaps in that knowledge.

UNCERTAINTY FROM THE PATIENT'S PERSPECTIVE

I have long been an advocate of shared decision-making and see the replacement of the paternalist or authoritarian model as an important ethical step forward in medicine. But personal experience showed me that shared decision-making is a mixed blessing for patients. As I have come to realize in dealing with my prostate cancer and MS, shared decision-making imposes burdens on patients that did not exist when paternalistic medicine was in force.

Shared decision-making assigns more responsibility to patients, and that responsibility can be hard for patients to handle. I now know from personal experience that when doctors share their uncertainties about treatment and the future, treatment decisions become more difficult for patients. And, as the example of breast cancer and my own experience with prostate cancer illustrate, medical and treatment advances often end up increasing the complexity of those decisions.

Illness has taught me that true shared decision-making requires much more than a discussion of the medical facts. It requires doctors to use their knowledge, training, and expertise to help patients understand the ways that different treatments could affect their well-being, values, and plans for the future. And shared decision-making requires doctors to help patients manage the uncertainties associated with many treatment choices.

Let me illustrate this with my own experience. In the case of my prostate cancer, I believe I should have been better informed about the medical controversies over whether to test and whether to treat. In retrospect, I wish I had known more about these debates. When my doctor recommended the PSA test, I didn't know that some experts questioned whether the test actually saved lives. I know now that it can detect cancer earlier, but it cannot show how aggressive that cancer will be. It might seem obvious that earlier detection would save lives, but that may not be the case. As I mentioned earlier, prostate cancer is most often a slow-growing cancer that men will die with, rather than die from.

I also needed more information about the benefits of watchful waiting as a treatment option. Good shared decision-making would have involved a discussion with my doctor about the psychological challenges of choosing watchful waiting and about ways to cope with those challenges.

Good shared decision-making would have involved a franker discussion of incontinence and impotence, too. These are unsettling topics for physicians and patients alike, but they need to be explicitly addressed. Few prostate cancer patients have considered what it would be like to be incontinent and impotent. Patients probably need more help exploring these topics than any other aspect of their decisions, but my own doctor did not explore them with me at all. Indeed, I believe he understated their actual incidence, which probably made it easier to avoid the exploration that should have taken place.

My doctor seemed reluctant to discuss incontinence not just before cancer treatment, but afterward, too. I went through over a year of extremely unpleasant and often embarrassing incontinence before he finally admitted that it was unlikely to get any better. And, based on my Internet searches, the profession as a whole seems unwilling to confront this element of prostate cancer treatment. How patients deal with these side effects should be an important area of study, yet my exploration of the literature uncovered little material addressing it, and even less that was helpful. Once I was dealing with incontinence, I tried without much success to find material about treating it. I recall no mention of the artificial sphincter that eventually helped me deal with this problem.

Before I made my treatment decision, I needed a fuller discussion of the possibility that my cancer treatment would leave me incontinent, and in particular of what it would be like to deal with it over the long term. Such a discussion would have helped me think more carefully about whether I wanted to accept surgery's higher risk of incontinence in exchange for the possibility of a longer life.

Much the same can be said about the issue of impotence. This, too, is a very common initial effect of the prostatectomy, but patients considering the surgery are simply told that in most cases the problem goes away over time. While I knew that there were drugs that could help patients who ended up with this problem, I never got accurate information about how frequently and to what extent they were successful in restoring sexual function.

Like incontinence, impotence was something I didn't know much about before I had cancer. My wife and I have adapted and been reasonably successful in maintaining a satisfying sex life. One accepts the situation because one has no choice in the matter, but there is still a serious sense of sadness and loss. Since incontinence and impotence are the two most serious side effects of treatments for prostate cancer, I believe I should have been helped at a subjective and personal level to understand what they would be like, even if that would not have changed my treatment decision.[5]

CONTINUING STRUGGLES WITH UNCERTAINTY

My experiences, as well as those of others in our cancer ethics group, show how hard it can be for physicians and patients to deal with uncertainty. On the positive side, members of our group did find that medical practice is different than it was in the old days of paternalism. For example, my doctors were quite open about the lack of good data on which prostate cancer treatment alternative produced the best survival rates. Several others in the group found their doctors similarly open about uncertainties in survival rates.

But our doctors seemed less willing to share uncertainty about treatment side effects. Some of our doctors downplayed the possibility that we would be left with side effects, and they rarely talked with us about what it would be like to live with those side effects. We are not sure why this happened, but have a few guesses. Perhaps our doctors didn't want to say anything that might discourage us from accepting treatment that could save our lives. Perhaps it is also hard for doctors to admit to patients (and to themselves) that their efforts to save patients could end up harming them, too. With prostate cancer, it could also be that doctors have a hard time being explicit about socially embarrassing matters like incontinence and impotence. My own doctors conveyed what I now believe was a false sense of certainty that I would escape the side effects of incontinence and impotence. And, once it was clear that I had not escaped them, some of my physicians remained reluctant to discuss them with me.

Our cancer experiences also show how patients struggle with the uncertainties surrounding their disease and its treatment. When I pressed my doctor to give me a clearer picture of what my MS symptoms would be and how quickly they would progress, I was asking for certainty where there is no certainty. And, although patients in our group understood many of the uncertainties associated with different treatment options, we were often unsure what to do with that information. Some of us ended up wanting a strong recommendation from our doctors because we felt unequipped to go forward on our own. Most of us also reached a point at which, in Leon Kass's words, "We held our nose and leaped." We had no idea where we would end up in the statistical pool, but we had to choose something.

Difficult though it was to cope with extreme uncertainty, I'm glad that I had an active role in choosing my cancer treatment. I would rather deal with the anxiety uncertainty produces than have a doctor in complete control of my medical care. Indeed, I wish my doctor had been more open about the uncertainty surrounding treatment side effects when I was making my choice. Doctors do patients no favor when they lead them to think that side effects are less likely than they actually are. Patients need a full and realistic picture of what life could be like for them both during and after cancer treatment.

Notes

1. Experts have developed a close monitoring approach that may be more appealing to men diagnosed with prostate cancer than watchful waiting has been. "Active surveillance" is an approach that "balances the desire to avoid treatment complications against the equally strong desire not to ignore a cancer—while at the same time minimizing the risks of overtreatment." Richard Hoffman and Steven Zeliadt, "The Cautionary Tale of PSA Testing," 170 *Archives of Internal Medicine* (2010): 1262–63.

2. Jay Katz, *The Silent World of Doctor and Patient*, 2nd ed. (Baltimore, Md.: Johns Hopkins University Press, 2002), 165–206.

3. As the next chapter illustrates, however, it is not always easy for patients to apply their values and preferences to decisions about medical treatment.

4. Dan Brock, "The Ideal of Shared Decision Making Between Physicians and Patients," *Kennedy Institute Journal of Ethics* 1 (1991): 28–47. Reprinted as "Facts and Values in the Physician/Patient Relationship," in *Ethics, Trust, and the Professions*, eds. Edmund Pellegrino, Robert Veatch, and John Langen (Washington, D.C.: Georgetown University Press, 1991).

5. Health policy experts are beginning to recognize the need to collect more information about patients' experiences with different treatments for diseases like prostate cancer. See Albert Wu, Claire Snyder, Carolyn Clancy, and Donald Steinwachs, "Adding the Patient Perspective to Comparative Effectiveness Research," *Health Affairs* 29 (2010): 1863–71. Such information would have helped me to decide which treatment option I preferred.

CHAPTER 5

Autonomy and Persuasion

Rebecca Dresser

Decisions about how to treat a newly diagnosed cancer are just the first of many medical choices cancer patients face. Another set of decisions arises as patients cope with the often brutal side effects and complications of treatment. For cancer patients diagnosed before the onset of debilitating symptoms, the treatment can feel worse than the disease. And for those already weak or in pain from their cancer, treatment can exacerbate the suffering. Cancer treatment creates its own risks and burdens, and patients and clinicians must make many decisions about how to manage that treatment.

In this context, medical decision-making is truly a process, not simply a one-time event. Patients undergo chemotherapy and radiation therapy over a period of months, sometimes years. During this time, they must decide how much pain medication to take, when to be hospitalized, and whether to interrupt a treatment regimen because the side effects have become too hard to take. Both the medical circumstances and the patient's preferences can change over time, as the anticancer drugs and radiation do their work. For the patient, the immediate burdens treatment imposes can begin to eclipse the long-term benefits it can deliver. In this chapter, I describe treatment management issues, focusing on a significant medical decision I faced.

A BAD DECISION

Before the radiation phase of my treatment for oral cancer, an oncologist and his resident explained the treatment regimen and its risks.

They told me that mouth sores and other radiation side effects would make it hard to eat and swallow. About half of the patients undergoing oral radiation require a gastrostomy feeding tube for adequate nutrition, they said. They showed me PowerPoint slides with photos and charts to illustrate their points. One slide was a photograph of a shirtless patient with a gastrostomy tube protruding from his stomach. The patient actually looked as though he was overweight, which made me wonder why the tube was needed.

By the time I started radiation treatment, I was already much thinner than the patient in the slide. I had lost some weight because my tumor made eating painful and laborious. The intensive chemotherapy regimen I had started six weeks earlier made it difficult to keep down what I was able to eat. Nevertheless, I was determined to avoid the feeding tube. To me, feeding tubes were involved with end-of-life issues. They were life-sustaining measures for patients like Nancy Cruzan and Terri Schiavo. I did not want to belong to that group of seriously ill patients.

I resisted the feeding tube for other reasons. Before my cancer diagnosis, I had been an exercise enthusiast and maintained a relatively healthy diet. I thought I was tough and wanted to show everyone that I wasn't one of the spineless patients who needed this kind of help. I was an overachiever, too. I did not want to become part of the bottom half (as I saw it) of any group I belonged to.

Control over my body and my life were also significant factors. I already had one foreign object in my body, a device called a port to deliver chemotherapy and simplify blood draws. The gastrostomy tube would be another unwanted physical mutilation. Treatment sessions, doctor appointments, and medication schedules had taken over my life, but eating and drinking were things I could still control. I would go to great lengths to keep from surrendering one more ordinary life activity to the world of medicine.

Tube placement would also require a few days of hospitalization. To me, the hospital was a dangerous place where I would be exposed to risky infections and might become the victim of a medical error. I would also be deprived of the security and relative comfort of my own home, stuck in a room with a stranger and probably a loud television.

Perhaps "chemobrain" (the mental fuzziness patients attribute to chemotherapy drugs) and the pain and antianxiety drugs I was taking also had something to do with my resistance. To be honest, though, I think my ingrained stubbornness and pride were the driving factors.

As I said at one of our bioethics and cancer group meetings, "You have cancer as you." Serious illness doesn't transform a person's character. Preexisting personality traits and flaws are part of the picture of how patients cope with cancer.

After a few weeks of combined radiation and chemotherapy, I was not doing well. At an appointment with one of my oncologists, we discussed what to do about my problems with eating and drinking. He said that we could try extra intravenous fluids and a few other measures that could help sustain me through the worst of the side effects. He also reminded me that the feeding tube was something to consider. But I was not ready for that, and wanted to try what I saw as the less drastic option. He agreed to this plan and wrote the necessary orders.

For another ten days or so, the doctors and nurses continued to cooperate with my quest to avoid the tube. Despite their efforts, I was continuing to lose weight and the extra fluids were beginning to produce their own side effects. Peter Joy, my partner and caregiver, wanted me to reverse my decision. Yet, I continued to insist that I could get through the ordeal without the tube. In a journal I kept during my illness, I wrote that the nurses were becoming concerned about fluid retention in my legs and ankles. This was my reaction: "I'm afraid they'll want to reduce the fluids, or use this as a reason for a feeding tube. But after today, I have only 11 more [radiation treatments] to go; I don't want to give up now!" As I became more debilitated, I became more determined than ever to assert my independence.

One day, however, I hit bottom. I was very weak and could barely get out of bed. Peter was frightened and declared that, despite my protests, we were heading to the cancer center. After we arrived, he took one of the nurses aside and begged her to persuade me to change my mind about the feeding tube. Taking one look at me, she agreed. By that time, I lacked the energy to argue with them. But what really convinced me to agree was the concern on their faces. I realized that I was facing a serious medical situation, and I gave in. My hospital admission diagnosis was "failure to thrive," a condition I associated with imperiled newborns, not someone like me.

In the hospital, I did have an annoying roommate with a loud television and a fondness for greasy smelling fast food. There were also a few irritating glitches in my care. (I was admitted right before a holiday weekend, which several of us learned is a terrible time to need medical care.) I was miserable, but no more miserable than I had been at home. And I escaped without injury. The tube insertion was a simple procedure, performed and followed up by a skilled and attentive staff. And the tube itself proved to be a blessing. I still had nausea and vomiting, but I was able to take in enough nourishment to maintain and then gradually gain weight. Tube feeding was simple, and the tube was easy to hide when I wasn't using it.

If I had accepted the tube earlier, I would have avoided a serious threat to my health and well-being. In refusing the tube, I had overestimated its burdens and underestimated its benefits. I was a relatively informed layperson, but I made a bad decision.

WHY THE REFUSAL?

Respect for patient autonomy is a major, if not the major, theme in bioethics. The field emerged at a time when patients and families were beginning to question the tradition of physician paternalism, in which doctors ruled over patient care. Bioethics introduced a new model of shared decision-making. In the new model, patients would have more control over their treatment. Physicians would continue to apply their special training and experience to determine patients' treatment options, but patients would decide which option they preferred.

Shared decision-making has become an axiom of contemporary medical education and practice. Yet, as Dan Brock describes in the previous chapter, the practice of shared decision-making doesn't always live up to the ideal. Few people want to return to the old days of medical paternalism, but the new regime is imperfect as well. My feeding tube story reveals some of the imperfections.

There are several ways to look at this story. One is to see it as an "all's well that ends well" tale. There were no long-lasting harms here. The clinicians treated me with respect and gave me the freedom to chart my own course. When that course became too risky, one of them convinced me to reconsider. Eventually, I replaced my bad decision with a better one. Agreeing to the tube was the decision most consistent with my overall goals, which were to complete the full course of cancer treatment and recover from the side effects as quickly as possible. And, while one could question my reasons for refusing the tube, they were understandable reactions to my situation. Indeed, some of my concerns were legitimate, such as my worry about being exposed to a hospital-acquired infection. Perhaps the decision process didn't go as smoothly or as quickly as one would like, but the basic model of shared decision-making worked in this case.

In hindsight, however, I wish that I had accepted the tube earlier. By the time I consented, I felt overwhelmed and wanted to quit cancer treatment altogether. (Fortunately, Peter and another nurse talked me out of that bad choice, too.) My delayed consent to the tube also imposed later hardships. It was a struggle to return from my emaciated state. Gaining weight can be as hard as losing it. Adding ten or fifteen pounds would have been easier than trying to regain the thirty I actually lost. Although my poor decision had no serious long-term effects, it did make my recovery more difficult than it would have been if I had accepted the tube earlier.

If shared decision-making fell short here, what was the explanation? One possibility is that I wasn't competent to make my own treatment choices. Oral cancer and radiation treatment are painful. I had a skin patch that was delivering increasing amounts of fentanyl, a powerful opiate analgesic. I was also taking antinausea drugs and an antianxiety drug to help me sleep. These medications definitely affected my cognition. About a week before consenting to the tube, I wrote in my journal, "I'm so out of it with the fentanyl that I have a hard time remembering things." (Reading the journal now, I can see that even my handwriting was affected. It looks cramped and shaky, as though I was too feeble to grip the pen tightly enough.)

Then there was the possible mental impact of the chemotherapy drugs. Although it didn't happen to every chemotherapy patient in our group, some of us believe the drugs affected our thinking. Simply trying to process the news that we had a life-threatening disease was distracting and disorienting, too. During treatment, we kept up with our work and other activities as best we could, but we were not completely with it. In our discussion, Arthur Frank mentioned that he had teaching and administrative responsibilities while he was undergoing chemotherapy. But he has doubts about how well he fulfilled them: "Why it was that anybody was taking me seriously on anything during this period, I don't know. Looking back, it was a total trip. I think of the whole thing as a long dream."

Medication and other factors can lead to fuzzy thinking, but they don't necessarily destroy a patient's decision-making capacity. Patients are legally authorized to make their own choices if they are able to understand the relevant facts about a proposed treatment—its risks and anticipated benefits—as well as the risks and benefits of any alternatives to that treatment (including the risks of treatment refusal). I don't think I ever lacked a basic understanding of the facts about the tube and what it could do. My judgment may have been clouded, but I believe I would have "passed" a capacity test. Indeed, if I was incapable at any point, it was when I was so weak and disoriented that I gave in to Peter and the nurse.

I think my treatment refusal is better described as an irrational medical choice. Dan Brock wrote about choices like this many years before we began this project. In a *New England Journal of Medicine* article,[1] Dan and a colleague described three forms of irrational thinking that can affect competent patients' decisions. In such cases, patients with the ability to make informed choices opt for a treatment alternative that fails to promote their primary goals and values.

One form of irrational thinking occurs when patients refuse a burdensome intervention that is likely to prevent later, more serious burdens. In refusing the tube, I was making this sort of choice. While I was preoccupied with avoiding the negative consequences of the feeding tube, I was exposing myself to greater harm in the form of extensive weight loss, dehydration, and a premature end to my cancer treatment. At the time, however, I was desperate to escape further assaults on my body. It seemed impossible that there could be a better life for me if I agreed to still another medical procedure. In the midst of my treatment, I lost sight of my overall goal of surviving the cancer.

The familiar phenomenon of denial can produce a second form of irrational treatment choice. Denial isn't always a bad thing for those facing serious illness. Without denial, cancer patients and their families would have a hard time getting through the day. But too much denial can interfere with good decision-making. Patients may engage in magical thinking, refusing to recognize the risks presented by certain health decisions. My persistent belief that I could tough it out without the feeding tube was a form of magical thinking. I ignored the increasing evidence that I was wrong in this belief. The severity of my condition was just too hard to accept.

Fear is a third phenomenon that can trigger an irrational choice. Sometimes patients are so afraid of the dangers associated with a medical intervention that they refuse to consider it. Patients gripped by irrational fear will not agree to undergo a procedure even when they recognize that doing so would be in their best interests. Looking back, I can see that I had an irrational aversion to the feeding tube. The implantation procedure didn't scare me much, but leaving home for the hospital and having a tube sticking out of my body did. In this case, though, the fantasy was much worse than the reality. I am grateful that Peter and the nurse pressed me to accept the tube.

What should happen when a competent patient seems to be under the influence of irrational thinking? Although it can be hard to detect irrationality, Dan and his co-author urged doctors to be on guard for its presence. Moreover, they wrote, doctors should speak out when they think patients are choosing irrationally. And, doctors should try to persuade patients to reconsider what appear to be irrational medical decisions. Thus, when a patient seems to assign too much significance to an intervention's short-term burdens, doctors should emphasize its longer-term benefits. When a patient fails to appreciate the risks of a treatment choice, doctors should present a frank and vivid picture of the harm that choice could produce. When a patient exhibits an irrational fear of an intervention, doctors should try to discover its origins and attempt to help her overcome it.

In my case, it was some time before anyone challenged my stance on the feeding tube. What explains this? Medical ethicist Jay Katz was a strong defender of shared medical decision-making, but he also knew that it is hard to achieve. Katz wrote that shared decision-making requires physicians and patients to engage in "probing conversation" in which conflict is inevitable. But this kind of interaction is a clear break from medical tradition. Doctors can be uncomfortable with the kind of discussion the model demands. Even today, few medical students learn very much about how to engage in what Katz described as "the give-and-take so necessary for joint decision-making."[2]

Perhaps out of a wish to avoid confrontation, my doctors cooperated with my efforts to avoid the feeding tube. Indeed, it was a nurse who took issue with my ill-considered choice. This was just one of several times when nurses reached out to me during a time of need. It was primarily the nurses who shepherded me through the ups and downs of therapy. And, at least twice, their objections rescued me from the consequences of a foolish decision. This was partly because they were in the right place at the right time. But perhaps the nursing profession's emphasis on care and compassion makes nurses comfortable with speaking up when they think patients are being unreasonable.

It is possible, too, that my position in the medical school had something to do with the doctors' deference. Several of my doctors knew that I taught medical ethics and worked with their medical colleagues. This might have made them hesitate to question or challenge my decision. The bioethicist-patients in our group were sometimes regarded as what Norman Fost called "honorary doctors," medically savvy people who needed less guidance than the typical patient. But this wasn't necessarily the case. Our professional status surely had its advantages, but we did not feel particularly well-equipped to deal with our cancer.

My deteriorating health status contributed to the situation as well. Before the start of radiation therapy, it was unclear whether I would need a feeding tube for adequate nutrition. At that point, the tube offered an uncertain benefit. But, as the radiation treatment progressed, my need for tube feeding became clearer. Although I knew that I was continuing to lose weight, I didn't appreciate how serious my condition had become. It would have been helpful for someone to say, "We've tried it your way, but it looks as though that strategy isn't working." Eventually, the chemotherapy nurse conveyed that message in forceful terms.

The fragmented structure of cancer treatment makes it hard for clinicians to see emerging big-picture problems in real time. Although I was making frequent trips to the cancer center, most of my visits were for chemotherapy or radiation treatment. During those visits, staff members focused on the specific task at hand. I saw the clinicians in charge of my overall care just once every three weeks. My precipitous decline occurred between those visits. Although I was receiving top-quality care in an institution where I worked and had personal connections—a privileged patient in all respects—it was Peter, my family caregiver, who called attention to the urgency of my situation.

STEPPING BACK

My cancer experience taught me how poorly prepared I was for making important medical decisions. Before I got cancer, I had been teaching and writing about patient autonomy, informed consent, and treatment decision-making for more than two decades. This background was useful, but not as useful as I would have expected. I knew something about patient psychology and the intricacies of medical decision-making—I had even read Dan Brock's article and talked about it with medical students and clinicians! But I never thought that I might become one of those irrational patients.

Making my own treatment choices was difficult and draining, and as this incident reveals, some of my choices were not good ones. Doctors writing about personal experiences with serious illness describe becoming confused and vulnerable when they became patients. Now I know that this can happen to medical ethicists, too. My academic and clinical bioethics experience was no defense against cancer's personal impact.

Accounts of medical decision-making often describe the patient's task as straightforward: Choose the treatment alternative that is most consistent with your values and personal circumstances. But this can be a complicated matter. We aren't experts in knowing how our values and preferences apply to situations we have never faced before. And no one teaches us how to make these decisions. As John Robertson observed in our discussions, "most of us are first-time players [with] no training." Despite this, when we are seriously ill, we are expected to make choices that can be among the most significant in our lives.

Our desires and objectives can conflict with each other, as well. I wanted to survive, but I wanted other things, too. I was unwilling to concede that my desires to avoid physical intrusion and hospitalization were incompatible with my goal of completing cancer treatment. I also inflated the threat the tube posed to my well-being.

In the previous chapter, Dan Brock discusses the difficulty of choosing among treatment alternatives when physicians and other sources convey conflicting information about potential outcomes. Patients face another kind of uncertainty when trying to predict their subjective responses to a treatment intervention. Patients cannot know how they will actually react to an intervention. I thought that a feeding tube would feel degrading and undignified, but I was wrong. I thought that being in the hospital would be horrible, but it wasn't that bad. I thought that the tube would be a major physical intrusion, but I later realized that my belief had been inaccurate.

My cancer experience also taught me that the cumulative physical and psychic assaults of treatment can begin to dominate a patient's thinking. In my case, this produced a reaction that Paul Appelbaum and Loren Roth wrote about in their classic study of why patients refuse treatment.[3] Some of the patients they interviewed refused treatment because they had "hospital fatigue syndrome." These hospitalized patients "were exhausted by their experiences and desirous above all of returning home." I was not in the hospital, but the intensive chemotherapy-radiation treatment I was receiving produced a similar kind of exhaustion. It was "treatment fatigue syndrome" that motivated my ongoing feeding tube refusal.

From a broader perspective, I learned that patients' choices emerge from a mix of ingredients and that not all of those ingredients are worthy of unqualified respect. There are individual values and individual "values." In the latter category are factors such as the childish stubbornness that contributed to my feeding tube refusal. In their study, Roth and Appelbaum found several patients whose treatment refusals reflected their "characterological style of dealing with stress." I suppose that stubbornness is my characterological style of dealing with stress. It is part of my authentic self, but it is not my better self. In this situation, it threatened to derail my desire to do everything I could to survive my cancer. It also threatened my more immediate desires for comfort, since dehydration and lack of nutrition were producing burdens more severe than the burdens of having a feeding tube.

Our cancer group discovered that an array of considerations affected our decision-making. We were not surprised that concerns about our loved ones affected our choices, but we were surprised at how complicated things can get. As Leon Kass commented at one of our meetings, "In the experience of illness, it is so often difficult to figure out what you want for yourself and for your beloved, precisely because what she wants for herself is so often shaped by what she wants for you." Less predictable considerations also affected our choices. For example, some of us had work and family connections to physicians advising on our care. We worried about offending them if we failed to follow their recommendations, and we made choices about how and where to be treated with those relationships in mind.

There are lessons for patients, family caregivers, and clinicians in what happened to me and others in our group. One lesson is that patient autonomy can be a challenging business. Even the most educated and savvy patients facing serious medical decisions may not be very good at applying their values and preferences to this new kind of choice.

Patients should recognize their lack of expertise and be more receptive than I was to what clinicians have to say. Clinicians may not share a patient's individual values, but they have seen many other patients in similar situations and can offer information on how other patients coped with interventions like feeding tubes. And, unfortunately, in today's overburdened health care system, patients may have to initiate this conversation. My case shows that even in the best settings, clinicians may not have a chance to get to it themselves.

Patients should listen to what loved ones have to say about their choices, too. Although illness and the treatment experience create fertile ground for interpersonal conflict, they also create opportunities for the best kind of care. Close family and friends know what is important to a patient and can provide a sort of "second opinion" on how the patient's values and concerns bear on the medical choice she faces. They may also have their own ideas about what decision would be best, ideas that have a legitimate role in patient decision-making. Patients should be willing to hear those views.

In addressing the demands of shared decision-making, Jay Katz described what patients must do to make the model work. He argued that patients have a duty to reflect on their initial treatment preferences. Patients should be willing to engage in conversation about their preferences, for such conversation can clarify confusion, correct mistaken ideas, and uncover irrational influences on treatment choices. Katz wrote, "the right to self-determination about ultimate choices cannot be properly exercised without first attending to the processes of self-reflection and reflection with others."[4] Consistent with this view, Art Frank's chapter on survivorship speaks of patients as "ethical subjects" with certain responsibilities in their relationships with clinicians and family members. Treatment decision-making is an ethical problem patients face, and there are better and worse ways to respond to this problem.

It may seem strange and in some respects unfair to impose duties on seriously ill patients. Why should people coping with life-threatening illness be expected to meet any ethical obligations? In *The Practice of Autonomy*,[5] Carl Schneider describes cases in which patients were too overwhelmed by illness and too intimidated by the medical system to take an active role in decisions about their care. This may be true for many patients, but not for all of them. Patients able and willing to play an active part in determining treatment should recognize that conversation and reflection are essential to making good medical choices. Inquiring, listening, and learning may not be things that we should expect of every patient, but based on my experience, they are appropriate to ask of some patients.

My case also adds weight to the argument that clinicians should respond actively when a patient's decision doesn't make sense to them. Questions like, "What is bothering you so much about the feeding tube?" and "Do you realize the risks you are taking in continuing to refuse the tube?" might have triggered constructive conversation about my changing medical situation. Clinicians should also engage in robust persuasion when patients are making what seem to be irrational choices. Some patients will not react well to this approach, but I think it is a risk worth taking. Patients are free to resist persuasion, but some of them will be glad, as I am, that a doctor or nurse provoked them to reconsider.

How far to take the challenge is a difficult question. Nothing in my experience or that of others in our group would support physically forcing an unwanted intervention on a competent patient. Nor would our experiences support the use of deception to induce patients to change their minds. But I do believe that what Roth and Appelbaum referred to as "coax[ing] and wheedl[ing]," as well as vigorous and persistent argument, can be appropriate. These are strategies we use to address disagreements arising in everyday life. They belong in the medical setting as well, especially when patients are making significant decisions about their care. Frank conversation and strong persuasion are essential to giving shared decision-making real meaning in the clinical setting.

My case serves as a reminder, too, that medical decision-making occurs over time. In many treatment situations, there will be opportunities to revisit an earlier decision after medical facts and personal circumstances have evolved. Our cancer ethics group discussed several instances in which patients modified an earlier choice, sometimes consenting to a formerly unwanted intervention, sometimes refusing one that had formerly been accepted. During a long treatment period, it is essential to keep the door open to new developments. Patients should feel free to alter an earlier choice that no longer seems right to them, and clinicians should give patients many opportunities to exercise this freedom.

Finally, some words on what caregivers can do when they disagree with a loved one's medical decision. As John Robertson describes in a later chapter, patient–caregiver negotiations require delicacy and diplomacy. Yet, sometimes, caregivers have to take command of a situation. In my case, Peter had to bully me into making an unscheduled visit to the cancer center. He had to plead with a nurse to join his campaign to convince me I should change my mind. In my case, these were good and necessary moves. I am glad that he contested my choice. In a sense, he was filling in for the clinicians who were unaware of my rapidly deteriorating condition.

Other members of our group reported incidents in which family caregivers alerted clinicians to a need for intervention. Based on our experiences, seriously ill patients depend on family and friends to act as advocates. Without a good advocate, busy doctors and nurses can overlook even the most privileged patient.

AUTONOMY REVISITED

Respect for patient autonomy does not require outright acceptance of every patient choice, but not all clinicians realize this. Some clinicians confuse shared decision-making with a no-questions-asked approach to patient choice (an approach Norm Fost calls "autonomy run wild"). Some lack the skills it takes to have a productive conversation about that choice, some want to avoid confrontation, and some believe they don't have time for what could be a long discussion. For whatever reason, it seems to our group that the patient autonomy movement has had the unfortunate consequence of inhibiting fruitful conversation about the choices patients make.

My feeding tube story does not support a return to medical paternalism. Nor does it support the use of coercion or deception when patients make bad treatment choices. But it does show that shared decision-making is easier said than done. In my case, even a well-educated patient and top-notch clinicians struggled to put shared decision-making into practice. And the fragmentation of modern medical care magnified the difficulties.

Before my cancer, I failed to understand how hard it can be for patients to determine the best way to exercise their decision-making authority. And I failed to understand how much patients can benefit from listening to the people involved in their care. As a cancer patient, I was not an isolated individual expressing a set of fully formed, preexisting preferences, but a student learning how to go about a new activity. I knew something about what was important to me, but I didn't know how to apply this to the feeding tube decision. I knew something about feeding tubes, but there were big gaps in my understanding. If I remain capable of make my own medical choices the next time I face serious illness, I hope I will be more engaged with others as I search for the right things to do.

Notes

1. Dan W. Brock and Steven A. Wartman, "When Competent Patients Make Irrational Choices," *New England Journal of Medicine* 322 (1990): 1595–99.

2. Jay Katz, *The Silent World of Doctor and Patient* (Baltimore: Johns Hopkins University Press, 2002), 96.

3. Paul S. Appelbaum and Loren H. Roth, "Patients Who Refuse Treatment in Medical Hospitals," *Journal of the American Medical Association* 250 (1983): 1296–1301.

4. Katz, *Silent World*, 124.

5. Carl Schneider, *The Practice of Autonomy: Patients, Doctors, and Medical Decisions* (New York: Oxford University Press, 1998).

CHAPTER 6

Volunteering for Research

Rebecca Dresser

For decades, the United States has made cancer research a high priority. Well before 1971, when President Nixon famously launched the "War on Cancer," the government established the National Cancer Institute (NCI) and invested millions of tax dollars in cancer research. Today, the NCI is first among equals at the National Institutes of Health. The NCI receives more funding than any of the agency's other institutes, and its director has more independence and budgetary control than does any other institute director.

The federal government is not the only source of financial support for the War on Cancer. Hundreds of nonprofit organizations raise money for cancer research, and private industry is heavily invested in developing new cancer therapies. Broadcast, print, and online media are full of reminders to support cancer research, as are airports, sports stadiums, shopping malls, and other public spaces. Our pluralistic and often divided nation seems united in its commitment to the search for better cancer treatments.

But money is not the only resource needed to meet this national commitment. A different type of contribution is needed from cancer patients. The quest for better cancer treatments generates a demand for human research subjects. Clinical trials are necessary to determine whether new approaches to cancer treatment give patients longer and better lives than standard therapies can provide.

Because novel approaches to cancer treatment must be tested in patients, cancer patients are often asked to participate in clinical trials. When and how should doctors present trial options to patients? What should patients understand about those options? Do patients have a duty to volunteer? Should there be national policies making trial enrollment mandatory in at least some circumstances?

In this chapter, I consider these questions in the context of my decision to decline participation in a clinical trial evaluating different treatments for my cancer. I made this decision for four reasons. First, I knew about the negative effects the trial could have on my care. Second, my doctor was honest about the downside of research participation and didn't question my treatment preference. Third, although I knew that my own treatment would be better because earlier patients had joined clinical trials, the trial seemed to demand too great a personal sacrifice. And fourth, although some say that progress against disease is so important that patients should be required to participate in research, under the current rules, I was free to reject the trial.

REFUSING THE TRIAL

After my oral cancer was diagnosed, a team of doctors recommended that I have chemotherapy and radiation therapy. I agreed to this plan, and then met with one of the doctors who would oversee my treatment. He was kind and informative. He took me to a computer and showed me a scan that revealed the dark mass threatening my life. I appreciated this effort. It was my tumor, after all; it didn't completely belong to the doctors. But he was the first doctor to recognize this. This doctor wanted me to understand what was going on in my body. His words and actions signaled that we would work together to counter this threat.

My doctor proceeded to go over the treatment plan, sketching a diagram and timeline describing what would happen. During the first six weeks, I would have two cycles of "induction chemotherapy" with four different drugs. The U.S. Food and Drug Administration (FDA) had just approved one of them, a biological called cetuximab, for head-and-neck cancer. One of the other drugs was also FDA-approved to treat this type of cancer. The remaining two had been approved to treat different forms of cancer but were used off-label to treat head-and-neck cancer. This means that the FDA has not determined whether the drugs are safe and effective against the kind of tumor that I had. Off-label treatments are common in cancer care and are covered by insurance if there is medical evidence supporting the off-label use. In my case, insurance would cover the off-label drugs because there was such supporting evidence.

After six weeks of induction chemotherapy, I would begin something called *chemoradiotherapy*. This would involve thirty-five days of radiation therapy combined with two or three cycles of chemotherapy (just one drug this time). My doctor warned that this intensive regimen would be rough. He said they wouldn't be recommending it if I were not relatively young, healthy, and able to tolerate the side effects.

He then said that there was another option to consider. His patients were eligible to participate in the "Paradigm Trial" comparing different approaches to treating the type of cancer I had. If I joined, I'd be randomly assigned to one of two groups. People in one group would have only chemoradiotherapy with one chemotherapy drug. People in the other group would first have induction chemotherapy involving three cycles of three chemotherapy drugs (three of the four drugs I would receive outside the trial). If their tumors disappeared after this, they would then have chemoradiotherapy with one chemotherapy drug. If their tumors still remained, they would have chemoradiotherapy with a different chemotherapy drug. He explained all this using another clear diagram. (As I write, I'm looking at the diagram and an online description of the trial. I could never remember the details on my own.)

It had already been a couple of weeks since my diagnosis, and I was eager to start treatment. The tumor was painful and the situation seemed urgent. I looked at my doctor and said, "I assume that enrolling in the trial would delay my treatment." He agreed that it probably would. I responded, "I suppose I ought to do this, but I can't stand to wait any longer to begin treatment." He looked at me and said, "I understand." And that was that.

A nurse later told me that I was just the second patient at the university cancer center to undergo the intensive regimen I chose. I was one of the patients getting cutting-edge treatment outside a trial. And, so far, it has been effective. Of course, I might have done well with one of the clinical trial regimens too, perhaps with fewer side effects. My intuitive sense was that four drugs plus chemoradiotherapy were better than what either of the clinical trial groups would receive. But perhaps I was wrong about that. Clinical trials often show that innovative treatment approaches are in fact not as good as standard therapies. It would take a rigorous clinical trial comparing the innovative regimen I received with other treatment regimens to determine whether my intuition was correct.

Patient advocates and the medical community repeatedly cite the need for more cancer patients to participate in clinical trials. They point to the pediatric cancer trial system as a model. Estimates are that about half of the children diagnosed with cancer receive treatment as part of a clinical trial. Dramatic improvements in childhood cancer treatment are the result, say research supporters, and the same thing should be happening with adults. But a much lower percentage of adult cancer patients participate in clinical trials.

As someone working in the medical ethics field, I was quite aware that clinical trials are essential to the development of better cancer therapies. By joining the trial, I would be helping with that process. And I knew that the regimen I was offered was available only because some of my predecessors had been willing to join similar trials. So, I knew there were good reasons for agreeing to participate in the trial.

Because of my background in medical ethics, however, I also knew about the potential personal costs of joining a trial. I knew enough to ask about the possibility of treatment delay, which is something most patients would never think about. I knew enough to understand that neither arm of the trial offered the full combination of chemotherapy drugs my doctor had offered. And I realized that neither group of trial subjects would receive cetuximab, the drug the FDA had just approved to treat my form of cancer. The popular perception is that clinical trial enrollment gives patients access to cutting-edge treatment, but I knew that this wasn't true in my case. As I understood it, the plan my doctor had originally proposed was actually the most innovative approach.

In refusing to join the trial, I must acknowledge that I put my personal interests above the interests of future patients. I must also acknowledge that I was better situated than other patients to understand the risks presented by trial participation. I must acknowledge as well that I received better therapies because other patients with my disease had participated in trials before I became ill. And I must acknowledge that some percentage of them did not realize, as I did, that trial participation might not be the best course for them.

RESEARCH CHOICES

The individual's right to refuse research participation occupies an honored place in modern research ethics. After the coercive Nazi experiments on concentration camp prisoners, the deceptive U.S. government-sponsored Tuskegee syphilis study, and an array of other research scandals, officials adopted rules aimed at preventing the abuse of human research subjects. The rules require researchers to obtain a person's informed and voluntary consent to study participation. Before enrolling patients as subjects, researchers must explain what will happen in a clinical trial, the risks and potential benefits of participating, and the alternatives available to patients who decide not to participate.

Today, researchers give patients invited to join trials consent forms with detailed study descriptions. Before asking for a patient's decision, members of the research team meet with the patient to review this information. Patients have opportunities to ask questions and discuss their options with researchers, physicians, and family and friends. Patients may not be penalized if they decide against joining a trial.

Yet, the elaborate system designed to promote informed choice succeeds only some of the time. Clinical trials are complicated, and consent forms are long and difficult to follow. Patients with a serious illness like cancer consider trial enrollment at an emotional time when it can be hard to focus on the material before them. Many people also lack background information about medical research that could help them make sense of the specific choices they face. Media hype about scientific breakthroughs contributes to popular misconceptions about research and the personal benefits patients obtain from trial participation.

For all of these reasons, patients make trial decisions with a limited and sometimes inaccurate grasp of the facts. Empirical studies show that sizable numbers of patients enroll in trials without a good understanding of the relevant information. The percentage of cancer patients who join trials believing they will receive the therapy that is best for them is troubling to people concerned with research ethics.[1]

Of course, I was not the typical patient invited to join a study. Instead, I was quite familiar with how trials worked. For many years, I had served on my school's Institutional Review Board (IRB), the committee that evaluates research proposals to ensure that they meet ethical and regulatory standards. I knew that the scientific and regulatory requirements associated with trials made them time-consuming and somewhat bureaucratic. I suspected that, if I agreed to consider trial enrollment, there would be more appointments, discussions, and paperwork before I could begin getting anything that could attack my cancer. That is why I asked the question about delay. And, based on my doctor's response, my hunch was correct.[2]

Few patients have the contextual knowledge about research that I had. And it's unlikely that anyone in the research setting will teach them what I knew. In all of my years reading about research ethics and reviewing clinical trials, I don't recall any mention of the need for doctors and researchers to tell patients that trial participation might lead to a later starting date for treatment. Some physicians may tell their patients about this possibility, but I doubt that many do.

Because of my background in medical ethics, I also understood the differences between the treatment regimen I would receive outside the trial and those I could receive if I enrolled. I knew that combining several cancer drugs often produced the best results in cancer treatment. And, thanks to my doctor, I knew I would get the most recently approved drug only if I chose not to join the trial.

As a patient receiving care at an academic institution, I also had opportunities many patients don't have. I was being treated at a leading cancer center where physicians were tuned in to the latest thinking about cancer treatment. My doctor was an academic oncologist with up-to-date knowledge of the therapeutic innovations relevant to my disease. The combination therapy he proposed was a novel approach that oncologists in less high-powered settings would be unlikely to offer their patients.

Enrolling in a clinical trial is often the only way cancer patients in less fortunate circumstances can gain access to an innovative treatment regimen. But the typical cancer trial offers patients only the *possibility* of receiving an innovative approach. Since trials usually compare newer therapies to existing treatments, some trial subjects will be assigned to groups receiving existing treatments. Trial enrollment gives patients a *chance* to obtain the latest regimen, not a guarantee.

For many cancer patients, the possibility of receiving an innovative treatment regimen makes trial enrollment worthwhile. But not all patients who want this option can get it. One member of our cancer ethics group encountered this problem. John Robertson's wife, Carlota Smith, was treated at a local cancer center. Doctors at the center participated in some trials, but none was enrolling patients with Carlota's specific type and stage of cancer. John now wonders whether he and Carlota should have done more to locate a suitable trial on their own, by searching the Internet or contacting an out-of-town cancer center. But, as John points out, an independent search for trials can be a daunting prospect for those dealing with all the other demands of serious illness.

Because I had very good health insurance, I was also free of financial constraints that limit other patients' choices. Some health insurers are reluctant to cover patients receiving cancer treatment through a clinical trial. Some won't cover innovative or off-label treatments. And relatively few uninsured patients have opportunities to enroll in cancer trials. Although uninsured people often enroll in other kinds of clinical trials as a way to obtain medical care, cancer trials tend to enroll well-insured and affluent individuals.[3] My care would be covered no matter what choice I made.

I was fortunate, too, to have a doctor who made no effort to "sell" the trial. By explaining the treatment plan before offering the trial, he made it clear that I was free to choose either alternative. Indeed, he seemed uncomfortable offering the trial and relieved when I said no. And his gentle demeanor was reassuring. I sensed that he would be there for me no matter what I decided. I doubt that every doctor is so supportive and even-handed, however, and those with strong personal or financial interests in boosting trial enrollment probably present the trial option more positively than he did.

In this situation, my doctor faced a classic ethical problem: the conflict between a doctor's fiduciary duty to his patient and the scientific demands of clinical research. Protecting and promoting the patient's best interests is the guiding ethical motto for physicians. According to the best-interests principle, doctors caring for patients should recommend the treatment that appears best for the individual patient. In traditional medicine, the individual patient's welfare takes priority over the interests of others, including the future patients who might benefit from what is learned through clinical trials.

But different ethical standards apply to researchers conducting clinical trials. Trials are designed to produce knowledge that could lead to better care for future patients. Although some patients in trials may end up receiving the intervention that is best for them, at the outset of the trial no one knows whether this will happen. Trials are not designed to deliver the best treatment to the individual patients who serve as subjects. To produce useful findings, trials must adopt rigorous scientific methods that are incompatible with an individualized approach to patient care.

Randomization is one research method at odds with the best-interests approach to patient care. Cancer trials typically assign patients randomly to one of two or more different treatment regimens. In randomized trials, the treatment a patient receives is determined not by a physician with the patient's best interests in mind, but simply by chance. But, according to traditional medical ethics, if a patient's doctor believes that a certain treatment regimen would be best for that patient, the doctor is ethically obligated to recommend that regimen. A doctor in this situation cannot in good conscience recommend that the patient join a clinical trial.

Not everyone thinks there is an irreconcilable conflict between patient care ethics and the scientific demands of clinical trials, however. Some say that doctors can ethically endorse trial participation if medical experts as a group are genuinely uncertain about the best therapy for a patient's condition. This state of affairs is called *clinical equipoise*. When clinical equipoise exists, there is a reasonable chance that any one of the available treatment approaches, including those being evaluated in a trial, will have the best outcome for the patient. Doctors who think a particular approach would be best for an individual patient may voice this opinion. But doctors should also acknowledge that medical opinions can be wrong and that research is needed to determine whether their views are correct. As long as clinical equipoise exists, appropriately humble doctors can preserve their allegiance to the patient's best interests while advising patients about clinical trial opportunities.[4]

Some research ethicists go further, arguing that clinical equipoise is not an essential ethical requirement in trials involving seriously ill patients. Although clinical trials are not designed to advance the patient's best interests, they say, trials are governed by ethical and regulatory standards that supply adequate protection to patients enrolled in trials. Trials are conducted primarily to generate knowledge, but trials must also be designed to minimize risks to the patients who serve as subjects. Moreover, trials may not expose patient-subjects to unreasonable risk. In trials evaluating different cancer treatments, every subject must receive some form of therapy. Doctors and researchers should tell patients when medical opinion favors a particular treatment approach, and they should make sure patients understand the differences between receiving personalized medical care and receiving treatment as a trial participant. But, even when clinical equipoise is absent, it is ethically permissible to give patients opportunities to join trials that will advance knowledge about their disease.[5]

I don't think the cancer center or my doctor would have offered the trial if there had been clear evidence that one treatment approach was better than the others. But I don't know whether clinical equipoise existed in my case— that is, whether the community of head-and-neck cancer experts was divided or unsure about which of the approaches I was choosing among would produce the best results for patients like me.

Clinical equipoise is not a straightforward standard, especially in cancer treatment. It can take many years to complete a cancer trial. For instance, data collection for the treatment trial I could have joined is scheduled to take seven years, and investigators will need even more time to analyze and publish the results. Innovations come quickly in cancer care, and promising alternatives may emerge during the years it takes to finish a trial evaluating older treatment approaches. Moreover, there are usually multiple approaches and combinations used against specific types and stages of cancer. Cancer treatment is a moving target, with numerous interventions in play at any given time. A systematic and up-to-date determination of where the community of experts stands on every alternative offered to patients as part of a trial or as clinical treatment seems impossible to achieve.[6]

Although I am uncertain whether clinical equipoise existed among the treatment options I was offered, I am certain that the Paradigm Trial met the requirements for ethical research—reasonable risk, the potential to generate valuable knowledge, and so forth. But, when I made my decision, I wasn't feeling altruistic enough to give up what seemed to be a superior treatment regimen to join a trial that I thought offered lower survival odds. I was not one of the patients for whom trial participation offered a clear opportunity for direct benefit. Entering the trial would require what seemed to me to be too great a personal sacrifice.

I also sensed that my doctor had a preference for the four-drug regimen. Perhaps I was wrong about this, but his choice to present that regimen first and his easy acceptance of my decision made me think I was choosing the treatment he thought would be best for me. Although he had agreed to recruit patients for the Paradigm Trial, in my case, he seemed to rank his commitment to patient care above his researcher duties.

I was not the only one in our group with a doctor who was less than enthusiastic about a clinical trial option. At one point in her treatment, Patricia Marshall became aware of a trial evaluating a drug she was taking and, thinking she ought to do her part for future patients, asked her oncologist whether she should enroll. Patty's doctor worked in a top-flight cancer center committed to research. But she did not want Patty to enroll in the trial. She explained that the trial would not be a good option for Patty because of the side effects she was experiencing. As Patty put it, "She wasn't thinking about me as a number, she was thinking about me as her patient who had side effects from an uncomfortable drug."

In Patty's case and in mine, two high-powered oncologists were unwilling to suppress their personal judgments about their patients' well-being. Our doctors seemed to experience a real conflict between research requirements and patient care. And, in both cases, they were less than enthusiastic about the research option. Other oncologists probably feel the same way, and if so, this is one likely reason for the low enrollment rates in adult cancer trials.[7]

These stories may be bad news for research advocates, but they show that the ethics of patient care remain a strong force for at least some physicians in cancer medicine. And Patty and I treasured this loyalty from our doctors. We knew that physicians' beliefs about optimal patient care weren't always correct, but we found it tremendously reassuring that our doctors appeared more concerned with protecting our personal well-being than with promoting research.

DO PATIENTS HAVE A DUTY TO VOLUNTEER?

Although I refused to join the Paradigm Trial, I was willing to make other contributions to the scientific endeavor. I agreed to have information about my case included in a clinical registry of patients with my disease. Registries compile data about the comparative success of different treatment regimens, but the evidence they produce is weaker than the evidence produced by randomized controlled trials like the Paradigm Trial. I also agreed to participate in two trials evaluating the long-lasting side effects of the therapies I received. The registry and trials carry small risks (to the confidentiality of my medical information) and inconveniences (the time it takes to answer questions about symptoms and the like). I'm happy to accept these risks and inconveniences to help doctors learn more about my disease.

The Paradigm Trial was a different story, however. I was frightened and wanted to have the treatment my doctor proposed first, the one I thought would be best for me. I exercised my autonomy and made an informed choice to decline trial participation. But was it ethical for me to choose as I did? Or, did I have a responsibility to enroll in the Paradigm Trial, particularly in light of my awareness that better treatment was available to me because patients had joined previous trials?

Some would say that I had such a responsibility. British philosopher John Harris is one of them. He and others believe that people have a moral duty to contribute to the common good, and this includes a duty to serve as a research subject.[8]

Harris contends that two ethical principles support a duty to participate in research. One, the beneficence principle, requires us to refrain from harming others and to act affirmatively to protect others from harm. For Harris, the duty to enroll in research is part of the duty to protect others. The principle of justice is the second basis of the duty to participate in research. People benefiting from earlier research advances owe a debt to the community, and they should repay that debt, Harris says, by participating in research to help future patients. People who fail to join studies are free-riders who unfairly benefit from the sacrifices of others. In Harris's view, the long-standing reliance on altruism as the basis for research participation permits, indeed promotes, an unjust situation.

Harris believes that the duty to participate in research applies not just to patients like me, who gain real benefits from past studies, but to everyone. He points out that nearly everyone will be a patient at some point, and anyone lucky enough not to need medical care will have relatives and descendants who do. Moreover, Harris notes, the knowledge that medical research is ongoing reassures healthy people that improved treatment could be available by the time they need it. In return for these benefits, he says, we should all be willing to serve as research subjects.

Harris stops short of endorsing a coercive research system. His primary aim is to convince more individuals to enroll in trials. Yet he also thinks a system mandating research participation could be morally justifiable in certain circumstances. At times, governments require individuals to compromise their personal interests for the sake of others. Some examples are mandatory quarantine and treatment of people infected by contagious diseases and mandatory jury service for most adults. According to Harris, research participation is another case in which governments might require some form of individual service to advance the interests of others.

People like Harris see medical progress as a social interest meriting the highest moral priority. This group believes in what ethicist Daniel Callahan calls the "research imperative," the principle that medicine has "an almost sacred duty to combat all the known causes of death."[9] In their view, ordinary people have an overriding responsibility to contribute to medicine's fight against death by serving as research subjects.

But this position clashes with the ethical judgments underlying research rules in the United States and other countries. According to the conventional view, research participation is praiseworthy, but in no way obligatory. Medical advances are important, but not important enough to support a moral or legal responsibility to enroll in research.[10] Those who believe research participation should remain voluntary say

the social interest in medical progress is less weighty than the justification for mandatory quarantine and treatment to prevent serious and
imminent harm to others. And they point out that jury duty requires
individuals to make smaller sacrifices than would a requirement to participate in most kinds of clinical research.

What would Harris and his compatriots think of my decision to
reject the Paradigm Trial? When my doctor presented the possibility
of trial enrollment, I was not feeling very grateful to the medical system.
My tumor was advanced, and I was facing a life-threatening situation
(I had been told that I had a 30%–40% chance of survival). I was frightened and desperate to act. Looking back, I think I was also angry that
my cancer had not been diagnosed earlier, when my survival odds
would have been better. In the months before my diagnosis, I had asked
three different clinicians about my symptoms, and none of them
thought it was anything serious. This failure of the medical system left
me feeling less appreciative than I might have been if a clinician had
made a more timely diagnosis.

On the other hand, I have benefited from research advances since
I was an infant, so I cannot argue that one instance of medical failure
exempted me from the moral obligation Harris describes. Thus, Harris
might label me a free-rider who unfairly benefited from the research
contributions of others. But perhaps I met my moral obligation by
enrolling in the clinical registry and the two low-risk trials related to
my cancer. Harris is unclear about the degree of risk individuals
are morally obligated to assume in research. Sometimes he seems to
have in mind only low-risk studies, such as those involving blood or
tissue donation. He suggests, too, that conscripting people to become
research subjects would be inappropriate "if the risks are significant
and the burdens onerous." At the same time, he does not completely
rule out a moral duty to participate under even these conditions. So,
my refusal to join the Paradigm Trial may have been indefensible in
Harris's eyes.

Others would have a different view of my conduct. As I said earlier,
the conventional research ethics position puts individual freedom of
choice above the need for medical advances. And although most of the
U.S. public is firmly behind the health research enterprise, relatively
few people take the trouble to respond to the many advertisements and
other publicity seeking to recruit study volunteers. At this point, most
people do not act as if they have a moral duty to participate. Because
individual freedom is highly valued in this country, it is even less likely
that the public would support a government program compelling

people to participate in research. A major cultural shift would be required for Harris's ideas to gain broad acceptance.[11]

Our cancer ethics group had a lively conversation about these matters. No one fully embraced Harris's ideas, but we all agreed that the quality of cancer care would be higher if patients like me had less freedom to obtain innovative therapies outside trials. Contrary to the position taken by many cancer advocacy groups, most of us thought it would be morally acceptable for policy makers to restrict patients' ability to obtain innovative treatments outside trials. Patients like me are not morally or legally entitled to receive the latest treatment regimens, particularly regimens whose safety and effectiveness remain unproven.

Thus, although we did not endorse the concept of a moral or legal duty to participate in research, we thought it would be fair for FDA and other government officials to make trial participation the only way for patients to gain access to promising innovative treatments with unproven safety and effectiveness.[12] At the same time, we recognized that certain patient protections would be required in a restrictive policy like this, such as strict requirements for clinical equipoise in trials comparing different therapies for treatable cancers.

RESEARCH OBLIGATIONS

I am not proud that I refused the Paradigm Trial. I am glad to be alive, though, and I don't know whether I would be if I had enrolled in the trial (especially if I had been randomized to the group that received chemoradiotherapy alone). I don't think I committed a serious moral violation, since neither the prevailing view of research ethics, nor the existing regulatory system, recognizes an affirmative obligation to participate in research. And, at this point, we don't live in a culture that expects people to make that sort of contribution to the general welfare. Relatively few people volunteer for research, and even fewer make the sort of personal sacrifice I was asked to make. Many who do make such sacrifices are probably unaware of what they are giving up.

My experience shows that cancer trials must be sensitive to the real situation of the patients who are asked—or expected—to enroll. Researchers and officials lamenting the low enrollment rates in cancer trials ought to focus on giving patients good trial options. Researchers seeking to enroll cancer patients should ensure they are making patients, in ethicist Nancy King's words, "a fair offer" supported by "good science and professional integrity."[13] In other words, they should worry less about the patient's research obligations and more about their own obligations, such as the obligation to protect seriously ill cancer patients from unreasonable risks.

Patients facing a serious threat to life want options that offer the best chance of successful treatment. Doctors and researchers owe them an honest and comprehensible explanation of the trade-offs involved in research participation. Well-informed patients are unlikely to choose trials involving treatment regimens that do not meet the clinical equipoise standard. And, they are unlikely to choose trials if their doctors seem unenthusiastic about that alternative. Moreover, not all oncologists offering trials will easily discard their ethical commitment to provide what they believe to be the best care for the individual patient.

I am grateful to the patients who joined trials contributing to the treatment regimen that has (so far) kept me cancer-free. I think they and all of the other patients who volunteer for research deserve strong praise for their willingness to help others. I would like to give back more than I have, too. If, in the future, I am asked to join another cancer trial, I will seriously consider doing so. But I would resist any effort to deprive me of the freedom to say no. And I suspect that most cancer patients would share my view. It is easy for healthy individuals to underestimate how onerous a requirement to participate in research could be for seriously ill patients. At the very least, debate over the duty to participate should expand to include the voices of people who have experienced serious illness.

Notes

1. For a review of the literature, see Nancy Kass, et al., "An Intervention to Improve Cancer Patients' Understanding of Early-Phase Clinical Trials," *IRB: Ethics & Human Research* 31, no. 3 (2009): 1–10.

2. I do not know how long the delay would have been. But because I was so desperate to start treatment, even a brief delay would have seemed unacceptable at the time. For general discussion of the bureaucratic impediments to conducting cancer clinical trials and how to reduce them, see Institute of Medicine, *A National Cancer Clinical Trials System for the 21st Century: Reinvigorating the NCI Cooperative Group Program* (Washington: National Academies Press, 2010).

3. For information on this situation, see Gerardo Colon-Otero, et al., "Disparities in Participation in Cancer Clinical Trials in the United States," *Cancer* 112 (2008): 447–54.

4. The classic discussion of clinical equipoise is in Benjamin Freedman, "Equipoise and the Ethics of Clinical Research," *New England Journal of Medicine* 317 (1987): 141–45.

5. For a defense of this position, see Steven Joffe and Franklin Miller, "Bench to Bedside: Mapping the Moral Terrain of Clinical Research," *Hastings Center Report* 38, no. 2 (2008): 30–42. Although patients in cancer trials typically receive closer monitoring and more attention than do patients receiving standard care, there is no clear evidence that patients in trials have better outcomes. For an analysis of comparative outcomes, see Jeffrey Peppercorn, et al., "Comparison of Outcomes in Cancer Patients Treated Within and Outside Clinical Trials: Conceptual Framework and Structured Review," *The Lancet* 363 (2004): 263–70.

6. Perhaps the closest approximation of such a determination comes from the National Comprehensive Cancer Network, which issues guidelines for treatment of different types of cancer based on systematic and ongoing review of the evidence by experts in the field. See National Comprehensive Cancer Network. Retrieved May 7, 2010, from http://www.nccn.org

7. For survey data suggesting that many clinicians put their duties to individual patients above their clinical research duties, see Charles Lidz, et al., "Competing Commitments in Clinical Trials," *IRB: A Review of Human Subjects Research* 31, no. 5 (2009): 1–6.

8. See John Harris, "Scientific Research Is a Moral Duty," *Journal of Medical Ethics* 31 (2005): 242–48.

9. Daniel Callahan, "Death and the Research Imperative," *New England Journal of Medicine* 342 (2000): 654–56.

10. Philosopher Hans Jonas was an articulate and passionate defender of this view. In a frequently quoted passage, he wrote:

> Let us not forget that progress is an optional goal, not an unconditional commitment, and that its tempo in particular, compulsive as it may become, has nothing sacred about it. Let us also remember that a slower progress in the conquest of disease would not threaten society, grievous as it is to those who have to deplore that their particular disease be not conquered, but that society would indeed be threatened by the erosion of those moral values whose loss, possibly caused by too ruthless a pursuit of moral progress, would make its most dazzling triumphs not worth having.

Hans Jonas, "Philosophical Reflections on Experimenting with Human Subjects," in *Philosophical Essays: From Ancient Creed to Technological Man*, ed. Hans Jonas (Englewood Cliffs, NJ: Prentice-Hall, 1974), 129.

11. For thoughts on convincing the public to make such a shift, see G. Owen Schaefer, Ezekiel Emanuel and Alan Wertheimer, "The Obligation to Participate in Biomedical Research," *Journal of the American Medical Association* 302 (2009): 67–72.

12. The Medicare program imposes such a requirement in certain circumstances. See Steven Pearson, Franklin Miller, and Ezekiel Emanuel, "Medicare's Requirement for Research Participation as a Condition of Coverage: Is It Ethical?" *JAMA* 296 (2006): 988–91.

13. Nancy King, "Benefits, Harms, and Motives in Clinical Research," *Hastings Center Report* 39, no. 4 (2009): 3.

CHAPTER 7

Resilience and the Art of Living in Remission

Patricia A. Marshall

Because we are alone with the alien thing that has entered into our self; because everything intimate and accustomed is for an instant taken away; because we stand in the middle of a transition where we cannot remain standing . . . the new thing in us, the added thing, has entered into our heart, has gone into its inmost chamber and is not even there any more, is already in our blood . . . [we] have changed, as a house changes into which a guest has entered.[1]

The experience of cancer can be so potent, so heavy with significance, that there is a radical and immediate shift in our awareness, an abrupt dissolving of what had been before to what is new and different. Cancer was that way for me. After going through cancer myself, then watching my husband, Larry Heinrich, die of this awful disease, I am not the person I was before.

The language of survival—and all that it implies—is often used to characterize living beyond the immediacy and urgency of cancer diagnosis and treatment, whatever form that living takes and however long it lasts. People say in a celebratory kind of way, "She is a Survivor!" Indeed, in our culture, a certain cachet is attached to being a cancer survivor. But we are all survivors in life, survivors through difficult times, through events of one sort or another. As the poet Mary Oliver observes, "Nobody gets out of it, having to swim through the fires to stay in this world."[2] It also seems to me wrong to use a term that elevates the lucky patients who survive cancer over those who do not.

I am much more comfortable with the language of resilience than with the language of survival. Resilience is what I want to claim, and resilient is who I am, as metaphor embodied. Being resilient does not have to be associated with being victimized by and surviving calamity or disaster. Resilience suggests to me a dynamic and transformative process empowered by hope, a posture in moving forward in life that is expressed and sustained in the very core of our being.[3] If we are fortunate enough to have the loving support of families and friends, and a strong spirit as well, we can be resilient. Resilience enables us to move beyond the cancer experiences that betray our bodies, leaving them scarred and wounded, and the grief that betrays our heart when we lose someone we love. Cancer fractures our courage and tests our endurance; resilience allows us to persevere in spite of the losses.

This chapter is about the art of being resilient and the process of recovery. I begin by describing cancer's double entry into my life. In our cancer ethics group of seven, I was the only one who both had cancer and cared for a loved one as he died of cancer. Then I tell the story of my mammogram one year after the death of my husband and two years after the end of my cancer treatment. After that, I explain what life has been like in the months and years after my two cancer encounters: the fatigue and other lingering physical effects of cancer treatment, and the grieving that has made all these things harder to bear. Cancer and grief cause visible and invisible changes; for me, the unseen ones have been the most difficult to weather. I close with my thoughts on the transformative power of resilience.

MY TWO CANCER STORIES

In the fall of 2005, I was diagnosed with breast cancer after a routine mammogram. This came out of the blue, for I had not felt a lump or noticed anything else unusual about my breast. Things happened quickly. A week after the mammogram, I received an urgent phone call to follow-up with an ultrasound scan. One day later, I had the scan, which showed a suspicious mass. A week after that, I had a needle biopsy that indicated a tumor. My radiologist told me that I had "your average, garden-variety form of breast cancer."

One month later, I had my first surgery. A surgeon performed a lumpectomy and removed eleven lymph nodes from my left arm. The diagnosis was stage two breast cancer. My second surgery had to be postponed when I developed an infection at the site of my first surgery.

I was treated in the emergency room and hospitalized with a two-inch wound in my breast. This event was a low point in my cancer treatment. Larry and I had to pack the wound with gauze soaked in saline solution. We did not know how long it would take for the wound to heal from the inside out. It added another element of uncertainty to our expectations. Fortunately, I was able to have the second surgery in about a month. Shortly after surgery, I had the first of what would be eight rounds of chemotherapy. And then I had six weeks of radiation treatment.

By the time my treatment ended, in July of 2006, my bald head was beginning to have white fuzz. My chest was sore, scarred, and burned from radiation. I gained twenty pounds during treatment, not an unusual occurrence. My body ached, and I was so very tired.

With time, my body began to heal from its wounds. But then cancer returned in a different guise. Ten months after the end of my treatment, my husband fell ill. We thought it was just the flu, but we were wrong. His symptoms became so severe that he was hospitalized. After eight days of tests, doctors diagnosed him with a rare and very aggressive form of lymphoma.

Larry died in July of 2007, just one year after I finished my breast cancer treatment. His illness was horrific. In a two-month period, he was hospitalized five times. Three times, he had to be taken by ambulance to the emergency room. He lost forty pounds, had to have many blood transfusions, and was put on all sorts of drugs. At one point, he was on such a high dose of prednisone that he became paranoid and delusional. Larry was lucid for less than half of this two-month period. He was in terrible pain, too. At the end, he was on hourly doses of morphine, but the pain still broke through. He had hoped to die at home, but his pain became so severe that we had to call an ambulance to take him to hospice in the middle of the night. He died five days later.

A few weeks before Larry died, he was in the hospital and I was home alone. Early that morning, I wrote something about what life was like at this time:

Death is standing outside the window looking in.
This is how it feels now. Up close but uncertain.
A strange duality of life. It's hard for me to say clearly what I feel.
Engaging in chemotherapy to push back this disease that is relentless,
that is taking over, that is claiming Larry's body that is no longer his.
In less than one month.

Imagining hope. For time. For a little bit of time.
There is never a good time. Now is not a good time.
We do not choose our time. We cannot.
Yesterday morning helping Larry shower.
His skin hanging from bones that I can see, that I can feel.
He has lost more weight. His body is deconstructing,
Dismantling. Revealing the core.
Revealing. Our conversations essential now. Urgent.
About the fundamental stuff.
I love you. I am sorry. I forgive you. You are forgiven. Thank you.

The intensity of the last two months of Larry's life was overwhelming. Two of my sisters, Mary and Jan, were with us most of the time. Our son Jeff and his wife Melanie, as well as our daughter Christy and her partner Amy, were able to stay with us for several weeks. I could not have gone through this without their help. I believe it would be impossible to go through such experiences alone, utterly impossible.

These two truncated accounts—of my breast cancer and my husband Larry's lymphoma and death—don't begin to tell the full story. They leave out so much, especially the love and caring we received from our family, friends, colleagues, and neighbors.

But my focus here is on the aftermath. The convergence of these two cancer episodes brought me to my knees. My recovery from breast cancer was totally eclipsed by my husband's illness and death. I realize now that my cancer recovery and my grief are forged together. Like two sides of a DNA strand, they were and continue to be inseparable. When life unfolds like this, unexpectedly and relentlessly, resilience is about the capacity to be both vulnerable and strong. Many times, resilience comes down to simply walking forward, with hands and heart open. It comes down to putting one foot in front of the other, even when the path is not clear. Perhaps especially when the path is not clear.

THE MAMMOGRAM TWO YEARS OUT:
A QUESTIONABLE REMISSION

My appointment at the Breast Cancer Center was scheduled for early on a Tuesday morning in October of 2008. I arrived on time and sat in the patient waiting area. A few other women were also waiting. I looked at them and thought, do they have breast cancer? Do they know they have cancer? Or are they here for just a routine mammogram? One woman had hair cut very short. It was gloriously white. I wondered if her hair was growing back now after chemotherapy. She seemed pensive. But was I just projecting onto her my own pensiveness, my own quietness in this liminal waiting space? I wondered, too, when I began to look at women with short hair differently—when I started imagining that they had traveled the same road that I am on now. I can't remember when I started to look at women differently. But I know that I do.

The nurse came out of the clinic area and looked around the room. Everyone in the waiting area turned to her, expectantly. "Marsha Brooks?" she called out.[4] The rest of us sat back, looking around, picking up our magazines or papers again. A man sat next to one of the women. They did not talk. He was crouched down low and his jacket hid part of his face. One woman, dressed in beautifully tailored slacks and a jacket, held her Blackberry in her hand. I watched her for awhile and noticed that she did not move her fingers. She stared at her hand and did not move, focusing her attention on what? Business-like, efficient, in charge. But, in truth, like the rest of us, waiting. Here, other people were in charge of us, managing our bodies, our breasts, and the machine that could pronounce us healthy or ill.

Eventually, the nurse called my name: "Patricia Marshall?" She went through the instructions—what to keep on and take off, where to put my clothes, how to wear the gown. I sat in another waiting area. An older woman sat across from me. We smiled at each other. That was all, an empathetic exchange in a place where strangers come together, women of all colors and backgrounds, wearing our gowns and our breasts; in these ways, we are not strangers. Once again, my name was called. The radiation technician who emerged from the mammography room was middle-aged and friendly. The patient who came out with her was smiling; she had had good news about her scan results.

The mammography room is small. It is dominated by the mammogram machine, sophisticated in its sleek and modern and angular lines. The technician had to move the platform up because I am tall. She was chatty and confident as she moved me into position, deftly rearranging my arm and my breast so that the image would be a "good" one.

My left breast was becoming smaller than my right one as I healed after surgery and radiation. It took a long time to get my left breast in just the right position. It was still tender around the pink and buckling scar. It hurt when the machine pressed hard against my skin. As the pressure grew, I grimaced in pain. Seeking relief, I stretched my neck and reassured myself that it would be over in only a few moments. I imagined my body protecting my breast, surrounded by loving hands, but this image was hard to maintain in the grasp of the rigid, utilitarian machine. I was thankful when my still intact right breast yielded more easily to the machine's pressure.

When she was finished with her work, the radiation technician told me to "hold on," that she would be back in a minute. I sat down on the chair that was put there for the women like me, women waiting to hear their fate. The lights were low, the edges of the room in shadow. It was very still. But my mind was not still. I was thinking about the work that needed to get done that day, about a meeting I wished I did not have to go to because I would rather be at home writing. I was thinking about Thanksgiving and where all of my visitors would sleep, about all of the trips I would be making in the next few months. My mind was busy with the stuff of everyday life.

Then the technician came back into the room and said that she needed to take another set of images. She was still smiling. And I wasn't worried, because this often happens. I was glad the radiologist could look at the images immediately and let me know the results. The technician went through the imaging process again, and I was in pain again, my poor left breast crushed by the mammogram machine.

And again, I waited. This time, though, I thought about my sadness during the last week. The man preparing the stone for Larry's grave had faxed me an illustration of his design. It showed vines on the edges of the stone, a fish (at Larry's request), Larry's name, and his dates of birth and death. The words, "Love, Kindness, Generosity" were at the bottom of the grave stone. I wondered if there would be room to put "Life is Rich!" there, too, because that is what I say all the time.

I also thought about what had happened two days earlier. It was October nineteenth, Larry's birthday. I was having dinner with some of my family, and we all raised our glasses to toast Larry's love for us, our love for him. I thought as well about the day before my mammogram, October twentieth. It was our anniversary. One of the beautiful things about love is that once you experience it—in whatever relationship—it is possible to experience it again. This is not a mystery, it is just a fact of our humanity and the potential that we have to be with others. What a gift I have been given—this crazy love of ours.

But then the technician came back into the room and said that she needed to take another set of images. She was more serious this time. After she left, I felt different. I began to think—to know—that the cancer had come back, perhaps in both breasts. I tried to imagine how

I would do it again, how I would manage work and chemotherapy and all that comes with breast cancer treatment.

It suddenly dawned on me that I should have asked someone to come with me to the center. It hadn't occurred to me that I might need someone to lean on while I had what I thought would be a routine test. I felt alone, so very alone. At that moment, I missed Larry terribly. How would I manage if my cancer came back? How could I possibly walk through that territory again without his support and caring? Immediately my mind shifted, and I began to get practical. I thought about what I would do, who I would need to depend on when I was sick or unable to take care of our rascal-of-a-dog, Mr. Bentley. My sisters and other family would help, of course, and all my friends and neighbors. But how much could I keep asking of others? They all have their own lives, their own busy schedules and families and work. And how would this affect my work? I was just beginning to catch up; now I would fall even further behind. All these thoughts and feelings rushed through me. I did not want to cry, though, I did not want to start to cry.

For the fourth time, the technician walked into the room. She still had a serious look on her face, and she still had a terrifying message. "One more time! Let's hope this time will be the last!" I looked at her and said nothing. I asked if she could get me a magazine to read while I waited. I looked at the recipes in the magazine but I could not see the words. I could only see what I imagined would be true.

Then there was a fifth time! The technician needed to do another set of images! By then, I was convinced that the breast cancer was back. I will be strong, I thought, I am strong. I have done this before. I hold my hands open in front of me. I am resilient. Still, in this tiny space of shadows and machine, my emotions took over. All I could feel was terror.

Finally, after what seemed like an eternity, the technician walked back in the room. This time, she was smiling at me, really smiling, not a polite half-smile. She said, "Good news!! You're all clear!!" I gave her a look of disbelief. I started to cry, and I couldn't stop. She said that she understood, that she had seen many former breast cancer patients suffer through ordeals like the one I had just been through. She thought I was crying because of the repeated mammograms and the good news, but it was a lot more than that. When she wrapped her comfortable big arms around me, I said, "I don't mean to cry! My husband died last year, and last week I got the fax showing what the cemetery stone will look like, and on Sunday it was his birthday, and yesterday it was our anniversary, and it doesn't seem possible that a year has passed!" And I couldn't seem to stop crying.

By then she looked worried, and asked if I was with someone. I said, "No, it just didn't occur to me." I asked if she could call my oncologist because I would surely be late for the appointment that was scheduled right after the mammogram. She said it was already taken care of, and she handed me the big manila folder with all the images inside so that I could give them to my doctor. Shaken but relieved, I got dressed. I walked out of the breast cancer center, through the hospital to the area where the oncologists see their patients, the same area where I had once had chemotherapy, holding the mammogram images close to my chest.

But I could not seem to stop crying. And, at this point, I didn't care if I cried. My tears bathed and comforted me. It did not matter what the strangers observing me thought, what stories they created for themselves about who I am and what I know and how I feel. I didn't want to see anybody I knew, though. I did not want to have a conversation with the doctors and other staff members who were my professional colleagues, because I did not want to reassure them that I was okay, that I would be fine, that this was simply a moment in time, a sacred moment in time. A border crossing of sorts. But I was back on the safe side. I was in remission, still.

BEING IN REMISSION

Treatment for breast cancer brings with it what I call an *Assault of the Trilogy*. You lose your hair, your breast is scarred forever, and you gain weight—all distressing changes for a woman. All three are physical evidence worn every day, on display. They remind you of cancer every time you look in the mirror, every time you get dressed. You see and feel a person who is you, but a different version of yourself.

By the time of the mammogram incident, I had my hair back. I didn't look like a cancer patient any longer, at least from the outside. But the mammogram was a sudden and vivid reminder of cancer's continued presence in my life. My treatment was supposed to be over, my tumor seemed to be gone, and it had been over a year since Larry died. Yet my body, mind, and heart had not recovered.

Even today, I live with lingering effects of the harsh treatments I went through. One persistent side effect is neuropathy from the drug Taxol, which was part of my chemotherapy regimen. Many patients experience neuropathy in their hands and feet, but it usually subsides over time. I still have neuropathy in my toes, however, and my neurologist says that it is unlikely to go away. In the beginning, the tingling sensations and numbness were painful. I'm now on a drug that helps with the pain, but the numbness remains. I also have muscle and joint pain from a drug I take to reduce the chance that my cancer will return.

My rheumatologist and my neurologist have been extremely helpful in treating these symptoms, but they've had a big impact on my quality of life. Because of the pain and numbness, I can't run ten-kilometer races the way I used to, and I don't walk with the same confidence I had before. I've learned to walk in a different and more cautious way than I used to, but I mourn the loss of the energy, strength, and stamina I once took for granted.

Recently, however, things have gotten a little better. Last year, I started to pick up the pace when I walked, and now I can jog slowly with my dog, Mr. Bentley. The first time I jogged two miles without stopping I was exhilarated. I took my shoes off, poured myself some bourbon and celebrated for all of us learning how to walk again, in a different way, but steady and sure! When you are in remission, patience and persistence can generate improvements even years after treatment is over.

Most disturbing of all are the hot flashes that began within a month after I started chemotherapy. Like all women on chemotherapy, my menstrual cycles stopped abruptly. Any woman who has had hot flashes will know what I mean. Mine were horrible; sometimes I would have more than twenty in a day. Hot flashes are quite simply torture by heat and water. Let me tell you what mine feel like. A volcano lives inside me, ready to erupt at any time. It begins with a warm sensation inside my body. Then it slowly burns outward, an intense heat that feels like fire spreading. If it's really bad, my entire body turns red—like the sunset peaking, like the color of Christmas, a red flush of extraordinary intensity. And I sweat. Sweat drips down my face, my neck, and my arms. My clothes are drenched. If I am standing, I sometimes feel faint and need to sit. At night, my sheets are drenched. It is not fun, although it can be funny. In fact, I would say hot flashes demand a sense of humor to survive them, and a very strong ego to stand up to them.

Those of us who experience intense hot flashes make jokes about having our own eco-systems. But that does not begin to address the serious impact that hot flashes have on a person's quality of life.

Sometimes I meet women who say they have never had a hot flash and I think, you are so lucky! My doctors have tried different treatments and, with their help and support, the hot flashes are not as frequent as they used to be. I'm fortunate to have a brother-in-law who is a breast cancer oncologist, and he has been a good source of suggestions for remedies to help with chemotherapy side effects.

The tiredness that I experienced after chemotherapy and radiation was unlike anything I had felt before. I spent many hours simply lying in bed, not reading, not talking, just lying quietly and still. The energy I put into caring for Larry during the two months he was sick, as well as the profound grief I experienced after he died, exacerbated the fatigue from my cancer treatment. Before all of this, I could never have imagined how tired I would feel.

There was also so much to do after Larry died. I spent an enormous amount of time taking care of the "business" of death and its aftermath. I thought I would be able to get most of it done in a month. How naïve I was! Even now, three years after his death, the work is still unfinished. And family life continues. With my own and Larry's large extended families, there are many birthdays and weddings and holidays to attend. And work goes on. Even to this day, I sometimes think, "I'm tired! Can I please just have a moment, a day, a week off?"

People reading this might wonder why I have not been more careful about setting limits. This wouldn't be easy for me. Family and work feed my soul. Also, it has never been more clear to me that I am alone now, and that I need the financial security that work brings. I am so privileged to love what I do, and to have family and friends who embrace and care for me.

The physical aggravations are bad enough, but they aren't the worst of cancer's long-lasting damage. The mammogram episode forced me to recognize once again the fragility of my existence. I am exquisitely aware of my vulnerability to illness, of my undeniable mortality. I don't know how much time I have left. I still think of myself as so young. I still have so much to give. I have not even begun to give back what I could. Yet, I also think of myself in a different way since I had cancer, since I watched Larry die of cancer. Now I just think I'm going to die sooner than later.

I'm not alone in feeling this way. Everyone in our group understands how I feel, and most of them share my outlook. Even Norman Fost, who downplays his cancer diagnosis, considers it an ongoing threat. At one of our meetings, he called cancer "the beast in the jungle,"[5] and said, "We're all concerned more or less that there's something lurking out there, namely cancer cells, and they're hiding. One day they're going to jump out again and bite us and kill us."

I no longer assume that I will have years of life ahead of me. I also can't do as much as I used to. I have always tried to do too much, and now I can accomplish even less of what I want to do. But I haven't accepted this yet. At one of our meetings, Dan Brock spoke of adjusting to the fatigue caused by his multiple sclerosis. It took some time, but he was eventually able to "cut himself some slack" at work. He came to accept the demands imposed by his illness, and accept that the world would be fine if he didn't publish quite as many articles as he did before. But I am still struggling with this. It is hard for me to admit that I cannot be as productive in my post-cancer life.

IN REMISSION WITH OTHERS

I've described some of the ways that life is different for cancer patients in remission—the fragility, the uncertainty, the losses. People who have been through cancer know all about these things, but those who haven't faced cancer, or something similarly terrifying, don't fully appreciate the damage cancer leaves in its wake.

Some of the people who lack that appreciation are members of the health profession. Once you are in remission, you spend less time in the medical system than you did during treatment, but you spend much more time in that system than most people do. You are watched more closely than other people are, and every scan, test, and doctor visit is a reminder that you are still in jeopardy. But it's surprising how often you run into clinicians who don't seem to know, or don't seem to care, how nervous you are when you see them.

One of my doctors is very good at taking care of medical problems like hypertension. But this doctor gets impatient when I complain about my aches and the hot flashes, saying that lots of women who have had breast cancer don't seem to have the problems that I do. Comments like this are not helpful because they diminish the importance of symptoms that patients experience and they shut down an opportunity for healing.

The technician who gave me all of those mammograms wasn't completely insensitive to my situation, but she was nevertheless surprised at the intensity of my emotion. She knew that I had had cancer before, and she must have known that I was frightened. But she didn't do much to comfort me as I went through the agony of those five mammograms. It was only at the end, after I started crying, that she reached out to me.

Rebecca Dresser had a similarly harrowing experience at one of her follow-up visits. A doctor was reviewing her latest scan, a scan that the radiologist had said was "clean." A nurse was at a computer taking notes, and the doctor told her he saw "something" on the scan. Rebecca was sitting right there, but the doctor didn't even look at her. When she worked up the courage to ask what he was seeing, he answered, "There is something there, but the question is what—is it cancer or is it something related to the radiation treatment?" He said he wanted to discuss the scan with the radiologist who had written the report. Then he walked out of the room, leaving the nurse to deal with Rebecca's panic. It took several calls and several days to confirm the radiologist's original opinion.

Once you have heard the bad news of cancer, you fear that you will hear it again. And that fear is rational, for you may indeed hear that news. But surely there are ways clinicians can help patients deal with the anxiety of follow-up visits. The technician handling my mammograms could have said something about what was going on, or the radiologist could have stepped in to give me a little information. The message might have been unsettling, perhaps words like, "We see a shadow that probably isn't anything, but we need to look again." Unsettling, yes, but better than waiting in silence, with only my horrible fantasies to occupy my thoughts. And Rebecca's doctor could have checked with the radiologist privately about the irregularity he saw; he didn't need to speculate about it in her presence.

I'm not implying that all clinicians ignore the anxiety of patients in remission. Although I've had some negative experiences with medical professionals; I've had many more positive ones. My breast cancer surgeon was terrific. My oncologist welcomes me with open arms; she knows what it means to be a healer. I trust her expertise as a physician, and she listens carefully to my concerns. Larry's oncologist was steadfast in his support, never flinching from telling us the truth, but always compassionate. I call another clinician "my teacher" because of her insights and uncanny awareness of things I can do to help myself heal.

A cancer diagnosis begins a long-term relationship with the health care system. Cancer patients in remission remain tethered to the world of medicine, tethered to the world of cancer. With time, follow-up examinations and tests become less frequent, but they rarely come to an end. If our cancer ethics group is any indication, many patients are ambivalent about this situation. At our meetings, we discussed how we crave the reassurance that comes from the clean scans and normal test results, but resent our dependence and the power that medicine still exerts over our lives. We would like to leave behind cancer and all its tribulations, but we're afraid to cut the cord, to escape from the medical bonds cancer continues to impose.

Arthur Frank first wrote about becoming part of the remission society in 1991,[6] but only later became aware of the institutional arrangements that lead people to identify themselves as members of that society. When our cancer ethics group was discussing post-cancer life, Art said, "One of the ways the remission society is assembled is by calling people back in for scans that then require you to think of yourself as someone who is part of this group," someone who remains on the precipice of illness. I know that I'm not a "cancer conscript," that I'm free to reject the medical orders to show up for the mammograms and other follow-up tests. And I would much rather think of myself as having rejoined the ordinary, healthy society to which I once belonged. Yet my scars, my lingering fears, and my need for reassurance keep me tied to the doctors and machines that monitor my body.

INVISIBLE HEALING, SILENT GRIEF

I am a perpetual cancer patient in the medical environment, but it is different in the outside world. Most people seem to think that my cancer is "over" and expect me to be the person I was before. This is both a blessing and a curse. I don't want people to think of me as "the person who had cancer," or "the person whose husband died of cancer." I am much more than that. Yet, I don't want people to ignore these traumatic events, either. Cancer is a dimmer presence in my life, but it is still there and it takes over at various points—when I have my scans, when I see something that reminds me of Larry, when I hear that someone else has died of cancer. I don't want pity, but I do want people to recognize what I have been through. I want them to recognize that I have changed and that some things are still a struggle for me.

There is an invisible dimension to healing from cancer and from grief. It comes from the privacy, solitude, and quietness that are essential to healing. This kind of "invisibility" is not a bad thing, because it creates an opportunity to be reflective, to make friends with the truths about the dramatic changes that have occurred in one's life, heart, and body. But the invisibility is not all good, for invisibility makes it easy for others to be silent. Some people cannot bear to acknowledge another person's losses and grief, and others put time limits on how long it should take to get "back to normal." People stop paying attention to what you have been through, and that leads to loneliness.

Several months after Larry died, I attended a professional conference. Although I went to the talks and participated in the social events, it was hard to do. One night, after a reception, I returned to my hotel room and wrote about my crazy, tangled, raw emotions and how alone I felt in my grief:

> Four months now. Gone. It seems utterly impossible.
> My heart is buried, covered in a sadness
> that collapses onto the nothingness that is here,
> that was filled not so long ago.
> How? How is it that words still come out of my mouth
> sounding possibly sane when I am screaming
> and it is an echoed silence of a voice that I hear, my own, longing.
> How can people walk and talk and act so normal
> while I am standing on the edge of this vast canyon of grief,
> craggy sides, razor sharp.
> And I long to be, to be what? To be where?
> It is a strange feeling. This aloneness.
> It helps to talk. To say out loud, "My husband died in July.
> Not so long ago. These are early days. It was horrific.
> He died within two months of his diagnosis."
> As if I keep saying it, then surely it must be true.
> As if I keep saying it out loud, then surely it must be real.

It's been several years now, but as I write this chapter, I am reminded of the overwhelming strength it took to keep going in those months after Larry's death, to keep going while I was drowning in grief and still weighed down by the side effects and fatigue from my cancer treatment.

RESILIENCE

Resilience is about finding the way to the other side of a tangled web of pain and uncertainty. It is about grasping at branches in a forest that on some days seems impenetrable. It is about striving to understand and make sense of what has happened. Resilience is about the profound and dynamic force of transformation.

My cancer treatment was hard, but I know many patients who suffered more than I did. I was able to continue some of my work, including teaching a seminar for doctoral students at home. My work friends and colleagues were a constant source of support. Along with my family and other friends, they fostered my resilience.

Resilience is an affirmation of strength and endurance. When I was a cancer patient, I decided to do three things during chemotherapy. I placed a pitcher of water next to the coffee pot in the kitchen and I drank two quarts every day. I read poetry every morning. And, each day I made it though chemotherapy, I gave myself a gold star on the calendar (a friend at work contributed a packet of stars). I now wonder if this is something all of us should do more often, especially on days that we are burdened by our vulnerabilities!

One of my sisters says that vulnerability is our greatest strength and our greatest weakness. I think she is right. There is a liberation that comes with allowing ourselves to be vulnerable as we live through the suffering of illness and treatment, as we confront our own mortality and experience the dying and death of someone we love. At the end of the day, so many things are just not that important. Kindness is. And gratitude. And courage, as much as possible. And love, the most important of all.

Resilience is expressed in different ways. Events happen or plans are made that reinforce the foundation of support and love so necessary for resiliency. Toward the end of Larry's first hospitalization, the doctor called me at home to tell me that his body was riddled with enlarged lymph nodes. I knew what this meant. My sisters Mary and Jan were with me, and a close friend was there too. It was morning, and we were still in our pajamas. We huddled together in bed, drinking our coffee. Sober, alert, imagining what would come next. Our collective energy provided a reassuring strength, knowing we would face together whatever horrible reality was before us.

A few weeks before Larry died, our son Jeff, daughter Christy, and one of Larry's old friends built a ramp from the side porch down to the driveway. It was good, I think, for the kids to work, to do something tangible. Larry used the ramp just three times, twice on relatively good days when he was able to enjoy sitting in his wheelchair outside. The last time he used the ramp was in the middle of the night, less than a week before he died, when an ambulance took him to hospice. In truth, the number of times the ramp was used does not matter. What was significant was the process of building the ramp, the effort, the act of resilience in the face of what they knew would be certain death.

These examples of resilience demonstrate the importance and strength of social bonds that nourish and replenish our capacity to endure. Resilience builds on these memories. But there are also singular moments that display the force of resiliency. One evening, my sister Jan and daughter Christy were talking with me on the back deck. We thought that Larry was in his bed resting. At the same moment, we all looked into the house and saw that somehow Larry had managed to climb over the side arms of the hospital bed and make his way through the living room and dining room to the pantry by the kitchen. He was leaning against the bathroom door, naked except for the diaper he was wearing; his arms and legs so thin. In the dim light, his features were hidden. Jan said, "It's Gandhi! Look, it's Gandhi!" Larry had wanted to use the bathroom and was determined to make it there.

In hospice, my sister Mary and I stayed by Larry's bed while he was dying. In the middle of the night, the day before he died, we were awake, listening carefully to his breathing, holding his hands, talking and telling stories. We decided to say some prayers. We knew the words to some, but we forgot the words to others and then we began to laugh. We just couldn't help ourselves. We were laughing with Larry, who would have known the words, but of course he couldn't help us. He was already on his way. We were like small children, trying to cover up our laughter under the blankets. But we were "outed" by a nurse who came in and told us we were making too much noise and that we needed to "keep it down." We still could not stop laughing. Larry, I'm sure, was enjoying this scene. The absurdity of all of it was just too much. Earlier in the evening, the man in the other bed had died. Mary and I were with him, too. Our laughter was both a source and an expression of our resilience. I think God really doesn't care too much about laughter at moments like this. I prefer to think of our behavior as a joyous send-off to another life, and I hope that someone has the good sense to laugh with me when I am dying.

RESILIENCE AND TRANSFORMATION

Remission is an up-and-down existence. And although the intensity of grief lessens with time, it never goes away completely; it simply evolves. My body and soul are a landscape of remission and grief, with the sharp and weary marks of loss and the smooth contours of blessed healing. I have been too close to death, but I have been granted a reprieve. With this reprieve has come what Art describes as "an acute sense of what a gift life is."

Every day, I walk in gratitude. When I walk down the street, I smile and people smile back at me or speak to me. And I think it's partly because of how I position myself as I walk through the world. I hold my hands open as a way of showing how I want to be engaged and give back, in appreciation of the gifts I have been given.

I don't want to exaggerate the positives. Some of the people in our cancer group spoke of feeling reborn, but I have never felt that way. For me, it's more a feeling of reorientation in my body and spirit, a feeling that I am drawing on the strength I had before cancer and grief. I know what it is like to crash, to lose the foundation that once supported me. Resilience allows me to walk on in trust, in faith, in hope, knowing that I am not alone, knowing that I will fall again, but knowing that I will rise again, as long as my spirit is able.

Notes

1. Rainer Maria Rilke, *Letters to a Young Poet* (New York: Norton, 1934), 65.
2. Mary Oliver, "Dogfish," in *Dream Work* (New York: Grove/Atlantic, 1986), 3.
3. There is now an extensive literature on resilience. See, for example, A. Masten and M. Reed, "Resilience in Development," in *Handbook of Positive Psychology*, ed. C. Snyder and S. Lopez (New York: Oxford University Press, 2005), 74–88; Janis Loomis Romond, *Posttraumatic Hope: The Lived Experience of Bereaved Parents 4–10 Years After the Accidental Death of Their Teenage Child* (Proquest, AAT 3431693, 2010).
4. The name "Marsha Brooks" is a fiction, not the actual name of the person who was called in the waiting room.
5. The phrase comes from the title of a story by Henry James. Henry James, *The Beast in the Jungle and Other Stories* (New York: Dover Publications, 1993), 33–71.
6. This was in Art's book, *At the Will of the Body: Reflections on Illness* (Boston: Houghton Mifflin, 1991, 2nd ed., 2002).

CHAPTER 8

The Allure of Questionable-Benefit Treatment

Dan W. Brock

C ancer treatment is expensive. Much of the expense is justified—treatment allows thousands of patients to live longer
and better lives. But some cancer treatment offers patients
little prospect of benefit, and some treatment does more harm than
good. Patients are subjected to harsh treatment near the end of their
lives, treatment that makes them miserable and, at times, actually has-
tens their death. Questionable-benefit treatment also raises health care
costs for insurance companies and government programs like Medicare.
When this happens, other people pay a price. Premium costs and government spending go up, people unable to pay higher premiums lose
insurance, and dollars that might be used to pay for more effective
health care go to treatment that does hardly any good.

When the members of our cancer ethics group became patients and
caregivers, we were well aware of the harms that questionable-benefit
cancer treatments inflict. Yet, we still wanted aggressive therapies.
For the most part, our yearning for continued life trumped any hesitation stemming from our academic knowledge. As I discuss in this
chapter, the objective case for limiting questionable-benefit treatment
is strong, but the subjective desire to try such treatment can be even
stronger.

HIGH COSTS, QUESTIONABLE BENEFITS, LIMITED RESOURCES

We were a quite privileged and, in that respect, unrepresentative group of people facing cancer. Those who had cancer, as well as the cancer patients we cared for, had access to high-quality health care. We were relatively affluent, and our health insurance plans provided for generous coverage. Not once in our extended discussions did anyone mention a problem with getting needed services paid for by insurance. In my own case, I simply assumed that my treatment would be covered by insurance, which it was, and the same was true for the other members of our group. Arthur Frank lived in Canada when he had cancer, and although he got the treatment any other resident would have received, it was the best treatment available at the time. Some of us also had access to treatments that are unavailable to many patients. In her chapter on clinical trials, Rebecca Dresser describes having coverage for an innovative treatment regimen, and insurance covered a questionable-benefit treatment for Patricia Marshall's husband, Larry Heinrich.

Ours were hardly the experiences of many cancer patients in the United States. Millions of Americans lack health insurance and cannot pay for expensive treatment if they get cancer.[1] Millions more have insurance that is inadequate to cover the treatment costs of a serious cancer. This problem is likely to persist. Even after the 2010 health care reforms take effect, an estimated 16 million Americans will remain uninsured, and many more will be underinsured. For these individuals, cancer can lead to financial ruin. According to current figures, over one-half of all personal bankruptcies in the United States are related to health care costs. These bankruptcies are filed by patients with no health insurance and by poorly insured patients who couldn't afford the out-of-pocket costs of their care.[2]

Although cancer care has always been expensive, the cost problem is becoming more serious. During the past decade, drug companies developed new drugs to treat many cancers, drugs that share two important features. First, they are extremely expensive, often costing in the neighborhood of $100,000 per year. Second, studies evaluating the drugs show that their average benefit is just a few additional months of life. The figure varies a bit, depending on the cancer treatment in question, the cancer for which it is used, the stage of the cancer, and the particular study evaluating the treatment's benefit. But, overall, these drugs often don't do much, if anything, for the vast majority of cancer patients.[3]

In health economics and health policy, the most common way to measure treatment benefits is to use something called the *quality adjusted life year* (QALY). A QALY combines the two principal benefits that medical treatments provide—gains in life expectancy and improved quality of life. Quality of life is measured on a scale with zero equal to death and one equal to full health. Patients with advanced cancer usually live with uncomfortable symptoms and side effects that compromise their quality of life. So, for example, if a treatment extends a cancer patient's life by two years, but the patient's quality of life is rated at .75, the treatment's overall benefit would be 1.5 QALYs.

Unlike treatment benefit measures that apply only to single diseases, QALYs allow analysts to compare the benefits of treatments for different diseases. This means that QALYs can be used to set priorities for overall health spending. Health planners consider the costs and benefits of different treatments—their relative cost effectiveness—by comparing their cost per QALY produced. Many policy analysts think this is a good way to measure the relative value of different treatments for different medical problems.

In Great Britain, an agency called the National Institute for Health and Clinical Excellence (NICE) evaluates new treatments, including new drugs, for their cost-effectiveness.[4] Based on this information, NICE makes coverage recommendations to officials at the National Health Service (NHS) about whether it should provide the treatment to NHS patients. The NHS usually follows the NICE recommendations. In general, NICE recommends against covering treatments that cost more than about $50,000 per QALY. (Sometimes British officials bend the rules for cancer patients, however. Recently, NICE relaxed its usual limit to allow more expensive coverage for rare cancers whose treatment does not have a large budgetary impact.[5])

Since Great Britain spends less than half as much per capita on health care as the United States, there is no reason to think that their cost-per-QALY cap should also be ours. Policy analysts in the United States commonly adopt a more generous cost-per-QALY cap of $100,000. This is the same figure they use to evaluate the cost-effectiveness of health and safety regulations, like rules covering workplace safety.

But even with this higher cap, many new cancer drugs don't measure up. A treatment that extends a cancer patient's life by three months at a cost of $100,000 has a cost per QALY of $300,000, far in excess of a $100,000 limit. The actual cost per QALY is even higher, because patients have a compromised quality of life during their few months of extra survival. A number of the new cancer drugs have performed so poorly that NICE reviewers have recommended against coverage, and Britain's NHS has largely accepted those recommendations. One drug the NHS does not cover is Avastin (bevacizumab), which is used in the United States to treat many patients with advanced colon, breast, lung, and other kinds of cancer.

Yet, the coverage issues are more complicated than I have suggested so far. Studies show that, every so often, one of the new drugs does a lot for a patient. The figure I mentioned earlier—a few months of extended life—is an average benefit for patients receiving the drugs in clinical trials. Although plenty of patients receive little or no benefit from the drugs, some patients get much more than a few more months of life. Even though the average life extension may be just three months, the possibility exists for a much larger benefit. Of course, each patient hopes to be the one who gets a better-than-average result. Patients want to try treatments that have very low cost-effectiveness in the hope that they will be at the positive tail of the benefit curve. And, in the United States, as physician Atul Gawande points out, "We've built our medical system and culture around the long tail" of patients who beat the odds.[6]

Basic fairness questions lie beneath the number-crunching involved in coverage decisions. When insurance and government dollars are used to pay for costly treatments like Avastin, there is less money available to pay for health care that could do more good for more people. The urge to do everything we can to help advanced cancer patients is laudable, but it can lead to dubious spending choices. Other patients lose out when we spend money on questionable-benefit cancer treatments. These ethical costs are serious, and they are disturbing to everyone in our cancer ethics group.

WHY NEW CANCER DRUGS ARE BOTH EXPENSIVE AND IN DEMAND

One way to deal with the problems I have described would be to lower the price of questionable-benefit treatments. This is not likely to happen, for several reasons. One is the intellectual property system, which gives patent protection to companies that develop new drugs. The patent system gives a patent holder an exclusive right to market a drug for twenty years, although in practice the period is significantly shorter because the clock starts ticking before the drug reaches the market. Patent protection allows a drug company to put whatever price it wants on its drug, for no potential competitor can market it during this period. Without patent protection, potential competitors could easily undercut the price of the drug developer. Drug companies also have a defense for their high prices. New cancer drugs are usually expensive to develop. Companies say they could not invest the large sums necessary to discover and develop these drugs without an intellectual property system that allows them to charge high enough prices to recoup their investment. This is especially important when the potential patient market for the drugs is relatively small, as it is for cancer drugs used primarily by advanced cancer patients unlikely to live very long.

Government policies contribute to the widespread use of questionable-benefit cancer drugs. Medicare is the largest purchaser of cancer treatments in the United States, and Congress has so far refused to allow Medicare officials to use cost as a basis for excluding cancer or other drugs from coverage. Similarly, the U.S. Food and Drug Administration (FDA) doesn't consider cost when it decides whether to approve a new drug for marketing.[7] As a result, drug companies have no incentive to limit prices.

Private insurance companies are also willing to cover many questionable-benefit cancer treatments. Many companies simply follow Medicare's coverage decisions. Fear of bad publicity, together with pressure from doctors and patients, makes insurers reluctant to refuse to pay for drugs that might extend a cancer patient's life, however briefly.

Last, but not least, patients and doctors want access to questionable-benefit cancer treatments. Since most patients have health insurance coverage for cancer drugs, whether under Medicare, Medicaid, or private insurance, they have little incentive to consider whether the drugs are worth the price. Patients need only consider whether their out-of-pocket costs from deductibles or co-payments are worth the expected or possible benefits of the drugs. Since their costs are only a very small portion of the drugs' actual costs, a small possible benefit can be enough to make an expensive treatment seem worthwhile.[8] Such patients will often be willing to give last-resort treatments a try, unless they want to avoid the serious side effects that can accompany such treatments.

In turn, doctors have both financial and professional reasons to favor liberal use of questionable-benefit treatments. Many oncologists buy cancer drugs directly from drug companies and then give them to patients in their offices. The profits from doing so are often a substantial portion of their overall incomes.[9] And, according to traditional medical ethics, a doctor's first and foremost responsibility is to do whatever is in the best interests of the patient, without regard to costs. With the rising and increasingly unsustainable costs of health care, this tradition is being challenged. But it still influences how many oncologists care for their patients.

The combined factors are not good news for cost control. In making treatment decisions, patients have little incentive to weigh the true costs of their care against its benefits—health insurance insulates them from the true costs. Oncologists, too, have little reason to consider costs. They instead have incentives to provide any potentially beneficial treatments, no matter how small the benefit and how high the costs. Drug companies have monopoly pricing power to charge as much as they can get for their products. Public agencies and private insurers have limited power to negotiate lower prices with the drug companies. In this situation, it is hardly surprising that the new cancer drugs often fail to represent good value for money.

ARE QUESTIONABLE-BENEFIT CANCER TREATMENTS WORTH IT?

What is the best way to decide whether to pay for "last-resort" cancer treatments? Some analysts say that the usual QALY approach is not the right one to apply here. Instead, we should apply something called the "willingness to pay" standard. According to this approach, the value of a treatment depends on how much a potential user would be willing to pay to obtain it. We can assume that patients near death would be willing to pay nearly all their resources to prolong their lives (unless they have strong desires to pass on their wealth to a loved one or favorite charity). This means that we should assign last-resort cancer treatments high value even when they are expensive and offer only a small chance of benefit.

But a big problem with this measure of value is that it varies depending on the wealth of the patient in question. The willingness-to-pay approach implies that interventions have greater value when provided to wealthier patients than to poor patients. This judgment conflicts with the idea that all persons have equal moral worth, as well as the idea that access to life-saving treatment shouldn't depend on a person's ability to pay for it.

There is another problem with using the advanced cancer patient's willingness to pay to guide decisions about health care coverage. Patients with a limited life expectancy don't have many other financial demands to consider. As a result, such patients will be willing to use their resources to prolong their lives for even a short time. But this is not the right perspective to take when thinking about the kinds of treatment and services health plans should cover. The better perspective is to think about a person's spending over a lifetime. The resources that advanced cancer patients would be willing to pay to prolong life could have been used earlier in their lives to pay for things like education, housing, and raising children. It's unlikely that people would want to go without these important things so that they could pay for a high-priced, but brief, extension of life with advanced cancer.

So, the right perspective to take in applying the willingness-to-pay standard is to ask how people would want to distribute their resources among the various needs and goals they have across their whole lives. This perspective reveals the opportunity costs of devoting great resources to slight benefits at the end of life. A rational and equitable allocation of resources to health care across the lifespan would not rely on how much patients are willing to pay for low-benefit care when they are facing death. The willingness-to-pay approach, like the QALY approach, assigns low value to low-benefit drugs. Both approaches suggest that the British NHS is justified in declining to cover expensive, low-benefit cancer drugs, and that Medicare, too, would be justified in refusing to cover them.

HEALTH ECONOMICS AT THE PERSONAL LEVEL

Our project was not about health economics and health policy, it was about our experiences as cancer patients and caregivers. As medical ethics teachers, we all knew about the problems I have just described. Yet, this knowledge had little impact on how we thought about cancer treatment for ourselves and our loved ones. In this respect, we resembled most patients and families facing a potentially lethal cancer. Patients with decent health care coverage are unlikely to give much attention to the health economics, ethics, and other policy considerations bearing on that care. Most people don't really know much about these matters. And those who do know about them, like the people in our group, will be too immersed in their personal ordeals to care much about the big picture.

You might think that medical ethicists who make their living giving professional attention to these matters would be able to integrate them into their experience. As I noted at the outset, none of us faced significant limits on what care was available to us or those we cared for. So, I can only speculate about what we would have done if we had faced such limits. But I believe that going through cancer ourselves may at least have helped us to think more deeply about how we would have responded to such limits.

Our treatment choices suggest that we would not have been happy if economic considerations had limited our access to treatment. No one in our group seriously considered declining treatment in the face of a cancer diagnosis. Although some of us faced daunting statistics and potentially serious side effects, we wanted to fight the disease. Patty Marshall's husband, Larry, had the most serious cancer diagnosis; there was almost no chance that treatment would prolong his life. Nevertheless, he wanted to "go for it." John Robertson's wife, Carlota Smith, also faced dire odds, but she tried almost every treatment that doctors offered. Rebecca Dresser was told that treatment had a 30%–40% chance of success, and those odds were more than enough for her to accept a difficult treatment regimen.

My own cancer, prostate cancer, was relatively easy to defeat. Even without treatment, there was a good chance the cancer wouldn't kill me. This is a reflection of the fact that prostate cancer usually grows very slowly. A common saying about prostate cancer is that more men die with it than from it, although it is responsible for more than 30,000 deaths annually in the United States. "Watchful waiting," which involves monitoring patients closely and treating only those whose cancer advances, is an acceptable option for many men with prostate cancer.

But, like the others in our group, I wanted to do whatever seemed to give me the best survival odds. As a result, I chose a treatment with serious side effects. A patient's Gleason score is one of the main prognostic measures of how aggressive the cancer is and how fast it is likely to progress. My Gleason score put me in about the mid-range in terms of aggressiveness. My doctor strongly recommended treatment over watchful waiting, and I followed his advice. But it is quite possible I would have done well with watchful waiting.

Their training leaves doctors with a bias in favor of "doing something" for seriously ill patients. Urologists and oncologists who have seen patients die from cancer are probably especially prone to this bias. For most physicians, the untimely death of a patient, especially a patient who might have survived with treatment, is the worst outcome. Although doctors caring for patients with prostate cancer disagree about the best form of treatment—not surprisingly, urologists favor surgery and radiation oncologists favor radiation—most are inclined to recommend one of these interventions rather than watchful waiting, which seems too much like doing nothing. A similar mindset explains the widespread use of the prostate-specific antigen (PSA) screening test to detect prostate cancer, despite the lack of strong evidence that it saves lives.[10]

The doctor's bias in favor of doing something is matched by an equally strong, if not stronger, patient bias. I felt a need to do something when I was diagnosed with cancer, and I also felt it when I was later diagnosed with another serious illness. As I wrote in my earlier chapter, "Coping with Uncertainty," I have a form of multiple sclerosis for which no treatment has been shown to be beneficial. But the lack of proven therapies hasn't kept me from trying several unproven medications, on the off chance that one of them would help. And these medications were not cheap. One cost my insurance company about $15,000 for six months of treatment.

The urge to try treatments is especially powerful for patients with cancer. I know from my own experience that it is extremely difficult to have cancer and not do something to try to get rid of it. Even in the face of the AIDS pandemic, cancer remains the disease that most frightens Americans: We are all at risk for it, and there are just a few things we can do to reduce that risk. Moreover, cancer is associated in the public mind with a "bad death," a death accompanied by pain and suffering. In my own case, I probably felt a special urgency to act because I was set to begin a visiting scholar position in a different city three months after my diagnosis. Yet, I believe this was much less important than my general desire to get rid of the cancer. So, my guess is that patients are as responsible as doctors are for the overtreatment that occurs in prostate cancer.

I was facing what seemed to be a relatively treatable and curable cancer—I was told this was one of the best cancers to have, if you have to have cancer at all. Because of this, I never felt that my life was really in serious jeopardy. Nevertheless, I might have been upset if I had been told that my "treatment" would be watchful waiting, because it was more cost-effective than surgery and radiation. The others in our group facing cancers with higher mortality rates were in grimmer and more desperate circumstances than I. So, they would probably have been even more upset if they had been denied treatment on grounds that it was not cost-effective.

Some British and American cancer patients are in this situation. Well-informed British cancer patients are likely to discover, in this

Internet world, that Avastin is available to cancer patients in the United States and some other countries. They may also discover that Avastin is available to wealthy British cancer patients who can pay to receive care in Britain's private health system. In the United States, patients without health insurance, or with insurance that doesn't cover Avastin, are in a similar position to British patients who cannot pay for Avastin in the private sector. These patients have usually tried all other treatments and so will see Avastin as the only possible way to postpone death.

Evolutionary biologists tell us that the desire to evade death is a deep and powerful element of our psychology. Our own experience teaches this lesson more forcefully. In everyday life, we deny the inevitability of death; indeed, everyday life would probably be impossible if we did not do this. But when we are diagnosed with life-threatening cancer, it is difficult to maintain the denial. (This is not true for everyone. My mother lived for six years with lung cancer, far exceeding her predicted life expectancy. At some point during those six years, she "forgot" that she had cancer. Denial can remain powerful even in the face of a clearly terminal illness.)

For most cancer patients, however, death is at the forefront of consciousness. It feels as though little time is left and much still to be done, experienced, and enjoyed. (Despite far outliving her prognosis, my mother wanted more time and was never ready to die.) For those of us without the consolation of believing in an afterlife, death represents the inconceivable: complete and permanent obliteration. Near the end of a long and painful battle with cancer, life can become so hard that death is welcome. But for most cancer patients most of the time, the desire and will to live are intense.

The typical cancer patient's state of mind is captured in the economist's willingness-to-pay standard for valuing treatment. As the model suggests, people may be willing to pay everything they have for any treatment. And patients may be willing to try anything to postpone death, even if failure is practically certain and success would be a few months of not very pleasant existence. Even in these dismal circumstances, trying cancer treatment can seem a much better option than the alternative. So, patients try treatment even when they realize they could be condemning themselves to something worse than death. And families are in the same boat. Fear of losing a loved one to cancer can move them to plead for more treatment, even when the patient is ready to stop. As I point out later, people can change their views once they have a better understanding of treatment burdens and the low odds that they will benefit. But this understanding often comes only late in the treatment process, if at all.

Just as patients will tell the economist they are willing to pay all that they have for a small chance to briefly extend life, they will tell their physician they are willing to try treatment that has a small chance to briefly extend life. But just as the answer to the economist is the wrong one to guide health coverage decisions, the answer to the physician isn't necessarily the one that should guide treatment decisions. The patient's request for last-resort treatment could do more harm than good, and it could conflict with that person's settled views on what would be a "good death."

Moreover, even cancer patients who want Avastin might be willing to concede that it's reasonable and ethically defensible for health plans to use limited resources to pay for more effective treatments. This might seem unlikely, but Rebecca had an analogous response when invited to participate in a cancer treatment trial. Although she decided against participating because it would have delayed and possibly compromised the quality of her treatment, she conceded that it would have been fair and reasonable for her insurance company or the FDA to restrict access to the type of innovative treatment regimen she received. Similarly, patients in our group might have admitted that a refusal to pay for an expensive and low-benefit treatment like Avastin would be fair and reasonable, while at the same time resisting and possibly challenging that refusal if we wanted the drug ourselves. We can recognize a rule as sound health policy, yet oppose that rule when it applies to us.

Personal experience with cancer gave us a better sense of how life-threatening illness can change a person's view of what constitutes "reasonable" treatment. That is why even reasonable and ethical limits on care at the end of life can seem outrageous to patients, their families, and their physicians. In all likelihood, we would have wanted to try something like Avastin, even if we believed it was reasonable and fair for our insurers not to pay for this drug. To be sure, we might have felt selfish, guilty, and hypocritical for trying to get care we thought was justifiably excluded from coverage. But, like many patients, we probably would have been preoccupied with our personal fight to stay alive. In truth, our health plans did cover treatments that they could reasonably and fairly have decided not to cover, such as the innovative treatment regimen Rebecca received and the treatment Patty's husband Larry received at the end of his life. The patients in our group who had access to such treatments wanted them.[11]

Of course, if we believed an expensive last-resort treatment could do us more harm than good, we might not have wanted it. But, even then, the powerful fear of death might have led us to pursue last-resort treatments against our better judgment. In his chapter on caregiving, John describes how difficult it was for him and his wife, Carlota, to refrain from trying one more ovarian cancer treatment. It took an emphatic statement by the doctor to convince them it would not be worth trying a treatment that could at best give Carlota a few months, months in which she would feel sick much of the time.

CAN WE SET LIMITS ON QUESTIONABLE-BENEFIT TREATMENT?

Some people are against setting any limits on end-of-life care, but they are probably a minority. Many Americans, if pressed, would probably agree that it is better to spend our limited health care dollars on treatments that are more effective than drugs like Avastin. And many would probably agree that if the costs are high enough and the benefits small enough, limits on end-of-life care can be reasonable and ethical. But can we realistically expect limits to be accepted by advanced cancer patients and their families? It is hard to know, for we have little experience with setting limits in our country. We can, however, look at how people in other countries have reacted to such limits.

Many Europeans see their national health systems as an important public good serving all members of the society. At the same time, they recognize that health resources are limited. The national health systems in most European countries are closed systems. This means that they can spend only a set amount of money on health care each year. In these systems, when patients are denied last-resort treatments, the money is used to meet the health needs of other patients. This makes limits on last-resort treatment more acceptable to European physicians and patients than to their U.S. counterparts. Because of our fragmented health care system, physicians in this country can rarely be confident that resources denied to some patients will be used for other patients who need them more. As medical ethicist Norman Daniels observed many years ago, this makes it harder for them to say no to their patients.[12]

Rationing is the allocation of a good under conditions of scarcity. When goods are rationed, some who want and would be benefitted by those goods will not get them. Limits on expensive, low-benefit cancer drugs are a form of rationing. Rationing is controversial in Europe, but people there live with it because they see the benefits of that rationing. Meanwhile, the American public remains deeply conflicted and inconsistent about rationing.

As I previously observed, although many Americans would probably accept limits on expensive, low-benefit interventions, even at the end of life, many others would probably reject them. Americans commonly claim that health care is not rationed in this country. It is, of course—people lacking health insurance are denied the same level of care that other patients receive. And, in reality, none of us gets every potentially beneficial medical intervention. For doctors, as well as private and government health plans, costs are a factor influencing patient care decisions. Despite this, many Americans insist that we are a rich country with no need to ration health care, especially if we can eliminate waste, fraud, and abuse in the health care system. When pressed to acknowledge the many places in which rationing exists in our health care system, they say that rationing care to patients facing imminent death would be morally wrong. The outcry about "death panels" in the 2009 health reform debate came from people holding this position.

This is not to say that Americans are completely opposed to controlling health care costs. Despite all the resistance to rationing, people are beginning to realize that the current rate of growth in health care costs is unsustainable. Controlling that growth and expanding health care coverage were the two central goals of the 2010 health reform legislation. Rising health care costs are becoming a personal problem for many Americans, as employers and insurers shift costs to individuals in the form of increased out-of-pocket payments. More Americans have also come to realize that rapidly rising health care costs are partly responsible for the small wage increases workers have received in recent years.

In sum, we Americans want to control the growth of health care costs, but we don't like it when cost controls apply to us or our loved ones. This resistance escalates in the presence of a dread disease like cancer. It is almost impossible to appreciate the persuasive policy reasons to limit expensive last-resort treatments when those treatments seem to offer the only escape from imminent death.

In the coming years, patients and their families will probably continue the quest for last-resort treatments, and the United States will probably continue to spend millions of dollars on poorly performing cancer drugs. It would be possible to prevent at least some of this spending. At the policy level, government officials could put into place an agency like NICE that rigorously evaluates new cancer drugs, and health plans could base coverage decisions on those evaluations. Is an American NICE likely in the near future? I doubt it; but the 2010 health reform law takes a step in the right direction. The law includes millions of dollars to support comparative-effectiveness research, and some of the money will be devoted to evaluating different cancer treatments. Such research will at least give health plans more systematic information about the relative value of expensive new cancer drugs.

Change could also come if members of the medical profession did more to help advanced cancer patients come to grips with their situation. Everyone in our group agreed that patients need to hear about the downsides of last-resort treatments from their doctors. Doctors must initiate the hard conversations that help patients understand the facts about such treatments. They must speak frankly about poor odds and poor quality of life. In short, they must discuss with patients and families the reality of impending death. As John and Carlota learned, there are compassionate and humane ways for doctors to deliver this message.

Doctors with the courage to have such conversations can protect patients from the hardships that come with the reckless pursuit of last-resort cancer treatments. But even the best of these efforts won't succeed in every case. Fear and denial will continue to drive some patients to seek treatments that have almost no possibility of helping them. The road ahead will not be easy.

Notes

1. For background, see Edward Partridge and Mona Fouad, "Community-Driven Approaches for Reducing Health Disparities in Cancer," *JAMA* 303 (2010): 1090–91.

2. See David Himmelstein, Deborah Thorne, Elizabeth Warren, and Steffie Woolhandler, "Medical Bankruptcy in the United States, 2007: Results of a National Study," *American Journal of Medicine* 122 (2009): 741–46. Cancer treatment costs are a problem all over the world. In developing countries, where cancer is a serious health problem, relatively few people have access to any cancer drugs. To date, "very little has been done to develop evidence-based guidelines for cost-effective cancer treatment or recommended therapeutic algorithms for use in poorly funded health care systems." David Kerr and Rachel Midgley, "Can We Treat Cancer for a Dollar a Day? Guidelines for Low-Income Countries," *New England Journal of Medicine* 363 (2010): 801–803.

3. Dan W. Brock, "Ethical and Value Issues in Insurance Coverage for Cancer Treatment," *The Oncologist* 15(Supp. 1) (2010) 36–42.

4. M. J. Buxton, "Economic Evaluation and Decision Making in the UK," *Pharmacoeconomics* 24 (2006): 1133–42.

5. National Institute for Health and Clinical Excellence. Citizens Council Report on Departing From the Threshold. Retrieved July 16, 2009, from http//www.nice.org.uk/newsroom/features/CitizensCouncilReport.jsp

6. Atul Gawande, "Letting Go," *The New Yorker*, August 2, 2010, 36–49, 45.

7. The FDA is planning to rescind its approval of Avastin as a breast cancer treatment based on newer studies showing a lack of effectiveness. In post-approval studies, the drug failed to give patients a statistically significant increase in survival, and some patients experienced serious side effects from the drug. The move is opposed by some patients and patient advocacy groups, however. Andrew Pollack, "F.D.A. Plans to Revoke Approval for Breast Cancer Drug," *New York Times*, December 16, 2010.

8. This situation could change. More insurance plans are adopting different payment requirements for some drugs, including questionable-benefit drugs. Some plans require patients to pay 25% or more of drug costs, instead of the usual small co-payment. In such cases, a patient's out-of-pocket costs can become very substantial. These requirements could thus reduce the number of patients who have access to questionable-benefit cancer drugs, but they would also make drugs with substantial benefits unavailable to patients who should get them. Thomas Lee and Ezekiel Emanuel, "Tier 4 Drugs and the Fraying of the Social Compact," *New England Journal of Medicine* 359 (2008): 333–35.

9. For background on this situation, see Mireille Jacobson, Craig Earle, Mary Price, and Joseph Newhouse, "How Medicare's Payment Cuts for Cancer Chemotherapy Drugs Changed Patterns of Treatment," *Health Affairs* 29 (2010): 1391–99.

10. For a discussion of these matters, see R.M. Hoffman and Steven B. Zeliadt, "The Cautionary Tale of PSA Testing," *Archives of Internal Medicine* 170 (2010): 1262–63.

11. Similarly, in the tax system, we typically take all exemptions and deductions to which we are legally entitled, including those we believe a just tax system would reject.

12. Norman Daniels, "Why Saying No to Patients in the United States Is So Hard," *New England Journal of Medicine* 314 (1986): 1381–83.

CHAPTER 9

Cancer Stereotypes

Rebecca Dresser and Norman Fost

The word *cancer* brings to mind terrifying things: death, pain, suffering, disfigurement. Cancer is "The Dread Disease,"[1] the affliction people fear more than any other. Cancer is insidious—it occupies the body without warning, often remaining unnoticed until it is too late. Cancer demands brutal treatment that intensifies patients' misery. Cancer sends people into battle; prevailing over cancer requires courage, spirit, and optimism.

These are stereotypes about what it means to have cancer. They hold true in many cases. Cancer often *does* mean death; indeed, it causes one in every eight deaths worldwide. Although cancer is not the leading cause of death in the United States, it comes in second.[2] Heart disease is the leading killer, but cancer is the more visible threat to the young and middle-aged. Everyone can see that there has been progress in treating and preventing heart disease, but improvements in countering cancer are harder to detect. And many cancer treatments *are* burdensome, inflicting pain and discomfort, sometimes killing the people they are supposed to help. Cancer often *does* feel like an attack that only the strong survive.

But the stereotypes don't always apply. The term *cancer* covers over a hundred different conditions. Although all involve uncontrolled growth of abnormal cells, each kind of cancer is distinct, producing different outcomes and requiring different sorts of treatment. Patients with the same kind of cancer face quite different situations, depending on the stage and grade of their disease. Cancer is not always that bad, and it is not always the worst disease a person can have. Cancer treatment can be relatively simple, and people don't have to be brave to recover from cancer.

Our cancer ethics group illustrates cancer's diversity. Our experiences reinforce cancer stereotypes, but challenge them, too. In the following section, Norman Fost tells his atypical cancer story.

THE CANCER OUTSIDER

I have always been an outsider. I chose bioethics as a career partly because it was a new ecological niche, one my medical school advisers had never heard of. And, in my bioethics career, I have always preferred to tackle previously unexamined issues and defend positions going against the stream. When Rebecca Dresser invited me to join a group of ethicists who had personally experienced cancer, I was pleased to be asked, but immediately felt like an outsider once again.

This was because I didn't think I was qualified to belong to this club. I didn't have "cancer" in the terrifying, life-threatening sense of the term. My cancer—a malignant tumor in my kidney—seemed to me to be cancer in only the technical sense of the word. As I wrote in my earlier chapter about diagnosis, I had the incredible good luck to have my kidney cancer detected quite early. The tumor was discovered because I had a medically unwarranted computed tomography (CT) scan during an emergency room visit for a kidney stone.

The sphere that showed up on this scan was technically a cancer, a malignant tumor. But my illness and treatment were not that big a deal. My cancer diagnosis produced a few weeks of worry, and I had to make some complicated decisions about which surgical approach, surgeon, and hospital would be best for me. But that was about it. My tumor was removed, and I am presumably cured. My treatment, follow-up, and likely prognosis were not much different than they would have been if the scan had revealed a cyst or a stone. My modest physical suffering was from a routine surgical procedure, not from the cancer. I do not feel as though I experienced "real cancer."

My encounter with cancer seemed utterly trivial compared with what the rest of the cancer group had experienced. What was I doing in a group that included friends who had experienced the prolonged suffering and death of a loved one, or the disabling complications of a mutilating operation? Perhaps this was a form of survivor guilt, but I didn't feel as though I had survived something profound or challenging. I felt like an impostor in the cancer ethics group.

My case illustrates the limits and hazards of labels and categories. "Cancer" can be anything from a basal-cell skin cancer to a metastatic brain tumor. Cancer treatment covers anything from simple surgery to intensive chemotherapy. Part of the public fear of the "C-word" is undoubtedly due to the inappropriate lumping of what are actually quite diverse conditions. My renal-cell tumor was cancer in anyone's lexicon, but it was trivial in my health history, less worrisome and less threatening than my kidney stones. My cancer seems more toward the "benign" end of the spectrum than the more dreaded end.

At the same time, I must admit that denial may be influencing my outsider self-image. There are comforts in seeing oneself as a cancer outsider. When I had the kidney tumor, doctors told me that the estimate for cancer-free survival in my case was 95%. Since then, however, I have read articles that put it substantially lower, at 70%–80%. My wife reminds me that aches and pains that might previously have been ignored now trigger a question—"Could this be it?"—that wasn't there before.

Thus, whether I like it or not, perhaps I *do* belong to the cancer club. My kidney cancer could come back to haunt me, presenting the sort of threat to my life that cancer is "supposed" to present. And, there is another thing that might make me a legitimate club member: my long-standing thrombocytosis. This is a bone marrow disorder that causes patients to have too many platelets in their blood. Like the kidney tumor, this disorder was picked up as an incidental finding in a series of probably unnecessary blood tests.

When I was treated for various medical problems through the years, doctors typically ordered standard blood tests that didn't add useful information about the illness of the day. But over time, these tests showed that my platelet count was slowly rising. At first, it was in the high end of the normal range. Over the decades, however, the counts doubled and then tripled, rising to numbers that could no longer be dismissed as within the normal range.

Eventually, I saw a blood specialist about the problem. He made the diagnosis of thrombocytosis, described treatment options, and recommended close monitoring for the time being. After a few years, however, I became what my doctor called "a platelet millionaire": my blood count had risen to a million platelets per cubic millimeter. This is four times the normal amount, and it is worrisome for two reasons. First, the increase in cell mass thickens the blood, which can lead to blockages in important blood vessels. This was a special concern for me, because I had yet another medical condition that elevated my risk of a blockage. Ten years earlier, doctors had discovered that one of the major arteries in my brain was unusually narrow. As a result, having too many platelets put me at serious risk of a major stroke. Second, the continued rise in platelet production signaled that my bone marrow was out of control, for reasons unknown. A bone marrow that overproduces one type of blood cell has a tendency to lose control of the other types of blood cells, including the white cells. People who have too many white cells have leukemia.

There it was again: cancer. This cancer was lurking in the future, a "beast in the jungle,"[3] the danger rising with every passing year. As a preventive measure, the specialist recommended daily hydroxyurea for the rest of my life. This might be the most trivial form of chemotherapy that exists. I simply take a pill each day, and the drug has almost no side effects. Like other chemotherapeutic agents, however, hydroxyurea inhibits cell production. In my case, it reduces the platelets my bone marrow produces, thus reducing my risk of developing leukemia.

So, I wondered whether this condition would qualify me for the cancer club. But, on reflection, I decided it did not. It seemed more like a genetic predisposition to a disease that might never manifest itself, rather than a disease state in itself. I wasn't sick. I was at risk for a fatal disorder, but so is everyone. I will probably die of something else before my bone marrow goes completely amok. In my view, admission to the cancer club requires something more than a runaway cell line. More suffering, more drug toxicity, more disability, more fear than I had experienced.

Then there was another development—my brain tumor. This was yet another incidental finding, picked up by unnecessary scans aimed at monitoring the cerebral artery problem I mentioned earlier. At first, there was just a tiny shadow that the radiologist didn't even notice. The next year, the shadow was bigger, and my doctor asked a couple of specialists to take a look. They said not to worry, that it was probably an aberrant vein. But then, like the platelets, it grew—too slowly to detect a change from one year to the next, but over the decade clearly growing. It was getting closer to the brainstem, which put me at risk of a heart attack and other serious problems. By 2009, the neurosurgeon no longer felt comfortable with watchful waiting. Like the platelets, it was only a matter of time before this tumor did me in. But this threat increased more rapidly than my blood problem did, and it was likely to cause trouble sooner than my bone marrow disorder would.

Now we're talking. A brain tumor. Brain surgery. This would be my ticket to the cancer club. But actually, it was not. My doctors assured me that the tumor was almost certainly benign, rather than malignant. They said it was probably something called a meningioma, which arises from the covering of the brain. Although meningiomas are not the sort of brain tumors people worry about, they are benign only in the microscopic world of the pathologist. Meningiomas can have very serious health consequences. From my vantage point, an expanding tumor destined to compress my brainstem was not "benign." If it pressed on my brainstem, it could kill me.

It turned out that the tumor was not a meningioma, but a different kind of "benign" tumor. But, even though it wasn't a true cancer, it was a much bigger deal to me than the malignant tumor in my kidney had been. Having the brain tumor removed required a more delicate, and more frightening, operation than the one to remove my kidney tumor. This time, surgery was a high-risk proposition. A temporary drop in blood pressure could reduce the blood flow in my middle cerebral artery just enough to cause an ischemic stroke, which could lead to serious brain damage or death. There was also a possibility of stroke from a blood clot, since I would have to stop my usual blood thinner for a week or so to prevent bleeding after the surgery.

But I made it through surgery in good shape, thanks to an excellent medical team and a bit of good luck. I was able to return to work and to my wonderful family. My "brain tumor" is gone, my kidney cancer is unlikely to return, and I am in "remission" from my disordered bone marrow. I probably won't die from any of my three "cancers," or nor am I likely to suffer in the way that others in the group have suffered from their cancer and its treatment. Although all three of my "cancers" would have killed me fifty years ago, today they can be kept at bay.

The truth is that my kidney stones and cerebral artery condition have changed my life in more profound ways than have any of my cancers. The kidney stones are extremely painful; every so often, they knock me off my feet. The condition that scares me the most, the one that most threatens my life, is the one affecting my cerebral artery. I understand the metaphorical problems with cancer. Cancer is invasive, it spreads and it destroys the body, which makes it ugly and scary. But the thing that I'm most likely to die from is this pencil-thin middle cerebral artery closing off, which could happen at any moment.

CANCER OUTSIDERS AND INSIDERS

Norm's experience doesn't conform to the popular image of cancer. His only true cancer—the kidney tumor—wasn't that serious. His cancer treatment was relatively easy to bear. For Norm, cancer is not the dread disease. What Norm dreads most is a health threat that has nothing to do with cancer.

Dan Brock's experience also doesn't fit certain cancer stereotypes. Like Norm, Dan told the rest of us that he felt like an imposter in our cancer group. Dan's prostate cancer surgery was relatively simple, and he considers himself cured. Although he has had to cope with long-term side effects of his cancer surgery, it is a separate medical condition—multiple sclerosis—that's had a much larger impact on his life. Like Norm, Dan's dread disease is something other than cancer.

For the others in our group, however, cancer lived up to its terrible image. Cancer was catastrophic for Patricia Marshall and John Robertson, depriving them of their beloved spouses in a relatively short time. After more than two decades as a cancer survivor, Arthur Frank no longer sees his cancer as life-threatening, but Patty and Rebecca (and perhaps even Norm) still live with the fear that their cancer will return. And, even though Art's cancer occurred a long time ago, it was for him a more difficult and life-changing illness than the heart attack he had when he was only thirty-nine years old. Some of the patients in our group also experienced the suffering commonly associated with cancer. Although Patty, Norm, and Dan never experienced any cancer symptoms, cancer was quite painful for Art and Rebecca.[4] Several of us also endured harsh cancer treatments that measured up to their notorious reputation.

None of us fits one cancer stereotype, though. In our group, there weren't any of the chipper, upbeat cancer patients journalists love to portray. Although we did what we had to do to deal with cancer, we weren't cheerful about it. To the contrary, we often felt depressed and defeated. Yet, for the moment at least, all of the cancer patients in our group are still around. Fortunately for us, it's a myth that people must be perky and courageous to make it through cancer.

In sum, cancer stereotypes can be inaccurate. Some of our experiences conformed to cancer stereotypes, some did not. But personal experience with cancer sensitized all of us to the power, and the downsides, of cancer stereotypes. Like other stereotypes, cancer stereotypes can do harm. In the remainder of this chapter, we describe our encounters with cancer stereotypes, as well as the damage such stereotypes can inflict at the personal, social, and policy levels.

CANCER STEREOTYPES—THEN

Cancer stereotypes have a long history. Two of the best historical accounts come from Susan Sontag and James Patterson. Sontag published her classic essay, "Illness as Metaphor," in 1978.[5] It is an eloquent and passionate critique of nineteenth- and twentieth-century cancer language and imagery. During the 1970s, when Sontag was a cancer patient, she saw how popular images of cancer increased patients' suffering and discouraged them from seeking the treatment that might save their lives.

Sontag thought that two cancer stereotypes deserved special condemnation. One was the notion that cancer patients are responsible for their disease. In the decades that preceded Sontag's essay, it was popular to describe cancer as an illness caused by repressed desires. According to this view, people who maintained a healthy attitude toward life didn't get cancer. Moreover, cancer patients who gave up hope were the ones who died; those with the proper will power could survive their cancer. Healthy people blamed cancer patients for their predicaments, Sontag wrote, which in turn intensified patients' suffering.

Sontag also decried the language of war that characterized cancer references. Cancer was an evil enemy; it was an invasion necessitating a brutal and dangerous counterattack. To be victorious against this evil enemy, society had to fight a war against cancer. Cancer was so evil that it became the politician's favorite metaphor for society's most terrible problems and calamities. Sontag denounced this sort of talk, contending that it stigmatized and demoralized patients. "The people with the real disease are . . . hardly helped by hearing their disease's name constantly being dropped as the epitome of evil," she protested.[6] Whether judgmental or demonizing, Sontag argued, cancer myths and stereotypes are bad for patients.

James Patterson's book, *The Dread Disease*, is a cultural history of cancer in the United States. Patterson examines popular conceptions of cancer from the 1880s to the 1980s, highlighting two competing images of the illness. One was promoted by an "optimistic anticancer alliance" that included doctors, scientists, and journalists.[7] The alliance portrayed cancer as a disease that could be conquered as long as adequate resources were devoted to research and early detection. Government officials became part of this alliance, promising to supply the dollars and scientific commitment that were needed. Patterson records the alliance's depressingly repetitive assurances that researchers were on the verge of major cancer breakthroughs, and that cures were sure to follow.

Although these overly optimistic pronouncements were useful in fund raising, Patterson believes they also contributed to a "cancer counterculture" skeptical of medicine's ability to prevail against cancer.[8] As the years passed, people saw little evidence of the significant treatment breakthroughs the alliance had promised. They saw family and friends suffering with and succumbing to cancer, and they remained terrified that this would happen to them. Patients who lost faith in conventional medicine often turned to the religious healers and enterprising charlatans who promised better results. Distrusting medical explanations of cancer, they persisted in thinking that cancer was contagious. And they criticized the "Cancer Establishment" for its wealth and its failure to produce meaningful progress against cancer.[9]

CANCER STEREOTYPES—NOW

When she wrote "Illness as Metaphor," Sontag expected the future to bring changes in cancer imagery. She predicted that once medicine had a better understanding of cancer, and more success in treating it, people would portray cancer more objectively, in terms that were less harmful to patients. Eventually, she hoped, cancer would be seen as "just a disease—a very serious one, but just a disease. Not a curse, not a punishment, not an embarrassment. . . . And not necessarily a death sentence."[10]

More than three decades later, we can see some progress in this direction. But there are still problems with the way society portrays cancer. Patients are still seen as complicit in their cancer, and military metaphors are rarely absent when cancer is the topic. Cancer metaphors are still common in political rhetoric, too, cropping up in speeches about evils like Islamic extremism, Mexican drug cartels, and the federal budget deficit.[11] Patterson's competing cancer cultures haven't disappeared, either. The anticancer alliance is still overly optimistic, and the cancer counterculture is as active as ever, offering quack remedies and simplistic explanations for why people get cancer.[12] The two cultures are in tension, but they each do their damage. Our group's personal experiences with cancer, together with public surveys and media reports, show that cancer fears and misunderstandings are still with us.

PERSONAL IMPACT

Stereotypes continue to shape individual perceptions of cancer. For much of the U.S. population, cancer is the most frightening disease.

In a 2004 survey, 42% of respondents said cancer was the disease they feared most, with heart disease second at 27%.[13] A 2009 cancer risk survey found cancer the top health concern of 37% of respondents, with heart disease at 21%.[14] In a 2007 survey, about 60% of the respondents reported that they "automatically" thought of death when they heard the word cancer.[15] About two-thirds of the people responding to a 2009 survey were concerned about dying of cancer; even more feared being in pain and having a poor quality of life due to cancer.[16]

Although the data are mixed, there is evidence that fear of cancer keeps some individuals from seeking medical care. In a 2007 survey of 500 cancer survivors, 13% of those who delayed seeing a doctor said they did so because they were afraid of what doctors might find. The actual number is probably higher, because this was a survey of cancer survivors. It didn't include people who failed to seek medical attention until their cancer was untreatable.[17] Some studies report that fear can also deter people from undergoing cancer screening tests like mammography. But fear can apparently push people in the opposite direction, too, for some studies find higher screening rates among people who are relatively frightened of cancer.[18] Fear could also explain why so many people are willing to undergo forms of cancer screening whose benefits are not clearly established.[19]

Before becoming patients and caregivers, everyone in our group thought it would be terrible to have cancer. Some of our cancer worries reflected what we had learned in our work, as well as what we had seen cancer do to relatives and friends. But our perceptions were undoubtedly shaped by cancer stereotypes, too. For example, when we learned of the cancer diagnosis, things like death, pain, and brutal treatment immediately came to mind. Once we had actual experience with cancer, we realized that some of our initial fears were unfounded. Cancer stereotypes gave us a distorted picture of our circumstances, at times creating stresses and sorrows that weren't supported by the facts.

Fear may have influenced some of the choices we made, too. When Art and Rebecca noticed what they eventually learned were signs of cancer, they dutifully sought help from their doctors. At first, they were told that their complaints were probably related to relatively benign medical conditions. Both were relieved by this response, but in retrospect, were too willing to accept it. It was news that they wanted to hear, because it wasn't news that they had cancer. Their responses contributed to delays in their cancer diagnoses.

Fear might also have made some of us receptive to overtreatment. In his chapters, Dan writes of his reluctance to accept watchful waiting as a medical response to his prostate cancer. Like many people with cancer, Dan wanted to "do something to get rid of it." Similarly, Rebecca refused to enroll in a cancer trial because doing so would prevent her from undergoing the more intensive treatment regimen her doctor had proposed. Their cancer fears may have led Dan and Rebecca to choose treatments that were riskier and more burdensome than alternatives that had a similar possibility of keeping them alive.

Even though we were well-educated and relatively knowledgeable, we made certain assumptions about cancer that weren't accurate. Some of our worst fears about cancer materialized, but some did not. Under the influence of cancer stereotypes, we made a few questionable decisions. In our group, cancer stereotypes contributed to unfounded panic and misguided choices as we dealt with the disease.

SOCIAL IMPACT

Although people today don't believe in a "cancer personality," people still search for cancer explanations. Nowadays, people don't associate cancer with repressed feelings, but with genetics, behavior, and environment. We ran into more than a few people who wanted to know why we had cancer. Presumably they wanted to hear that our disease was linked to a family history, behavior, or environmental exposure that didn't apply to them. There is comfort in the belief that coming from the right family and environment, and behaving in the right ways, will protect people from cancer. And the focus on cancer-causing behavior suggests that cancer and personal responsibility remain linked in contemporary thinking.

The belief that cancer patients are responsible for their recovery may be less popular now, but we saw signs of it when we were dealing with cancer. Many people encouraged us to "be strong" and to "fight." In *At the Will of the Body*, Art wrote, "During my heart trouble, no one suggested I fight my heart, but one of the first things I was told about cancer was, 'you have to fight.'"[20] Those of us with more recent cancer experiences heard similar statements. Although the people who made these remarks were trying to be helpful, they also seemed to be expressing their need to believe in patients' power over their disease. We see the same need expressed in the popular media, which rarely feature cancer patients who admit to feeling overwhelmed. Even stories about advanced cancer give prominence to patients who have every intention of defeating their cancer. The belief that patients have control over their recovery makes cancer less frightening to the "worried well."

But the persistent stereotypes make it harder for patients to deal with cancer. Patients shouldn't have to take on the role of instructor to healthy people unaware of cancer's complex and multiple causes. They shouldn't be burdened with explaining that genes, environment, and personal behavior can affect a person's chances of getting cancer, but can't fully account for why specific individuals get cancer. Patients shouldn't have to counsel healthy people about their cancer risks, nor should patients be expected to reassure others that they will be safe from cancer. Some patients may find it rewarding to act as cancer teachers and counselors, but for us, coping with cancer gave us more than enough to do.

The social pressure to maintain a positive outlook isn't helpful to patients and caregivers, either. The celebrities, public figures, and ordinary people embracing the happy warrior role can be irritating to people who know what dealing with cancer is really like. After going through cancer, the people in our group find the mandatory public optimism more offensive than inspirational. When patients facing terrible odds insist that they will prevail over cancer, they trigger our pity, rather than our admiration. We don't want to discourage optimism among the patients and families who find it helpful in coping with their situations. But patients and families should be free to express, and journalists willing to report, pessimism, too. Anger and sadness are part of the authentic picture of cancer.

Cancer stereotypes have another bad outcome for patients: shame and humiliation. People with cancer are less stigmatized than they once were, but stigma remains a problem. Even today, many patients feel they have become social outcasts. When Art was treated for cancer in the late 1980s, he felt he "had no right to be among others."[21] His bald head and intravenous line made it impossible to conceal his cancer patient status. If he appeared in public, he feared, "someday, somewhere, someone would see my bald head and scream, 'Oh my god, he has cancer.'"[22] Patty and Rebecca went through chemotherapy more recently, and they too felt embarrassed about their bald heads and other visible cancer signs. Before going out, they had to brace themselves for the stares they inevitably attracted. It was easier to hide out at home or at the cancer treatment center, places where they would be safe from scrutiny. Such reactions aren't unusual. Feeling stigmatized, patients opt for isolation at a time when they most need comfort and support from others.

Although cancer stereotypes can make life harder for patients, we have to admit that they aren't all bad. Norm writes of feeling guilty that his cancer wasn't as terrible as it was for others in our cancer ethics group. He wonders whether he belongs in the group, and whether he is worthy of the sympathy and good will that true cancer patients deserve. These remarks point to a bright side of cancer stereotypes. Sociologists write about the rewards of the sick role, and cancer patients surely enjoy many of them. As cancer patients and caregivers, we were the beneficiaries of immense, and largely unexpected, generosity. People didn't always respond well, but they often did. Many reached out to us, and they did so partly because we had the dread disease, cancer. Our circumstances were dire, warranting the best they could give.

The attention moved and sustained us—we will never forget it. But we don't want cancer to be the only disease that elicits such benevolence. When cancer stereotypes lead people to reach out in extraordinary ways, patients facing illnesses that are equally or more threatening may lose out. Cancer "exceptionalism" isn't fair if it results in less care and sympathy for seriously ill people whose conditions don't have the cultural clout that cancer does. Having dealt with both cancer and a serious "something else," Norm and Dan are particularly aware of this imbalance.

Cancer stereotypes have a few other positive effects. Besides triggering care and concern from others, cancer confers a certain stature on those who have dealt with the condition. As Art put it in one of our discussions, "It really wakes people up when you say, 'I've had cancer.'" This is especially useful for teachers like us. Students prick up their ears when we talk in our classes about being cancer patients or caregivers. When we speak with doctors and nurses about ethical problems in medical care, we have a sense that our views carry more weight because we have dealt with cancer ourselves.

The stereotypes also make cancer an effective excuse for relinquishing one's ordinary responsibilities. As we learned, cancer is about the best reason someone can give for seeking relief from work and other obligations. For the most part we "played the cancer card" only when we really needed to; indeed, we probably went too far in the other direction, pushing ourselves to perform when we should have been taking it easy. But, every once in a while, when we were tired or feeling down, it was nice to have cancer as the explanation for not showing up.

In the years since Sontag wrote, cancer patients have begun to resist the irritating and oppressive dimensions of cancer stereotypes. Through writing and other kinds of artistic expression, patients challenge—and ridicule—the dominant narratives about cancer, replacing them with more authentic and edgy accounts. Although no one would call our group radical, at times we engaged in our own small acts of resistance. When someone asked us how we were doing, we refused to say "fine," and instead told the truth. When someone told us how good we looked, we politely thanked them, but emphatically disagreed. We spoke openly about the difficult and disgusting parts of having cancer, and we told a few irreverent cancer jokes. Sometimes we simply lacked the patience to play by the cancer stereotype rules.

POLICY IMPACT

Cancer stereotypes influence policy choices. In this country, cancer's status as the dread disease gives it a special claim on health resources. We mention two areas in which cancer exceptionalism may be distorting health policy.

For many years, cancer has received the lion's share of government support for research targeting specific diseases. For example, in 2009 the National Institutes of Health awarded nearly $7 billion dollars to cancer research; infectious disease studies received about $4 billion dollars, mental health research about $2.5 billion, and heart disease research about $1.5 billion.[23] Plenty of people want the government to spend even more money for cancer research, including President Obama, who lost his mother to ovarian cancer.[24] Much of the public favors increased cancer research funding, too. In Texas, a state not known for backing big government programs, voters approved a 2007 ballot initiative authorizing a $3 billion bond sale to fund cancer research.[25]

Research priority setting is a complex matter, but one that merits ethical scrutiny. Choices about allocating research dollars should reflect public health needs, as well as the potential for progress in particular areas.[26] Cancer is certainly a serious public health problem, but so are lots of other conditions. It's not clear that cancer's position as the number one research target is scientifically or ethically defensible.[27] It's also debatable whether different types of cancer research receive defensible levels of support. Research aimed at improving cancer treatments is justified, for it could help many suffering patients in the future. At the same time, it's reasonable to ask whether research aimed at cancer prevention is adequately funded, for it too could produce valuable public health benefits.

These are just some of the hard questions that cancer research funding raise. We aren't equipped to answer them here, but want at least to recognize them. Although cancer treatment and prevention are things we care about, we don't want cancer to get more than its fair share of research dollars. We are uneasy at the thought that the research that helped us get through cancer may have supplanted research that could have helped people in even greater need. If cancer's status as the dread disease leads to research funding inequities, then this is another problem with the stereotypes about cancer.

Cancer stereotypes may be contributing to unwarranted cancer screening and treatment, too. Government officials and insurers rarely question the value of cancer spending, and their hesitation is probably related to cancer's notorious reputation. Like much of the public, many government officials see cancer as the worst disease. And they know that public perceptions make setting limits on cancer spending politically dangerous. Insurance executives also fear the negative publicity that comes from setting such limits. Meanwhile, as Dan describes in his chapter on last-resort treatments, doctors have professional and financial incentives to treat cancer aggressively. And, as we discovered ourselves, cancer's fearsome image leads patients to accept questionable cancer tests and aggressive treatment measures. Cancer stereotypes probably play a part in sustaining expensive screening programs and treatments with marginal health benefits.

PERSISTENT AND PROBLEMATIC STEREOTYPES

Like most important subjects, cancer is complicated. Although the stereotypes have some validity, they oversimplify cancer and are often out of date. People today have a better understanding of cancer than they did when Susan Sontag wrote *Illness as Metaphor*, but people still don't see cancer as "just a disease." And it's unlikely that cancer stereotypes will ever completely vanish. Too many people benefit from the stereotypes. Cancer's dread disease status promotes generous funding for cancer researchers and advocacy groups. Pledging support for anticancer programs is a vote-getting tactic for politicians. Dramatic media stories about cancer draw big audiences.

Although cancer stereotypes have a few upsides, patients and their families would be better off without them. It would be better if people could hear a cancer diagnosis without assuming it meant suffering and death. It would be better if patients and families didn't have to deal with the misperceptions and stigma that still surround cancer. It would be better if the public stopped treating cancer as an exceptional disease, and saw it instead as one of many serious conditions meriting attention and concern. Cancer stereotypes may appear benign, but they can be malignant.

Notes

1. In 1971, when he announced his support for a stronger federal commitment to cancer research, President Nixon referred to his goal of "conquering this dread disease." James T. Patterson used the term in his well-known cultural history, *The Dread Disease: Cancer and Modern American Culture* (Cambridge: Harvard University Press, 1987), 249.
2. American Cancer Society, Cancer Facts and Figures 2010. Retrieved September 2, 2010, from http://www.cancer.org
3. This phrase comes from a Henry James story. Henry James, *The Beast in the Jungle and Other Stories* (New York: Dover Publications, 1993), 33–71.
4. Art vividly describes his cancer pain in *At the Will of the Body: Reflections on Illness* (Boston: Houghton Mifflin, 1991, 2nd ed., 2002), 22–35.
5. Susan Sontag, *Illness as Metaphor* and *AIDS and Its Metaphors* (New York: Picador, 1990).
6. Sontag, *Illness*, 85
7. Patterson, *Dread Disease*, ix.
8. Patterson, *Dread Disease*, ix.
9. Sontag railed against with both extremes: the "bromides of the American cancer establishment, tirelessly hailing the imminent victory over cancer," as well as the skeptics focused on the lack of real progress in cancer treatment. Sontag, *Illness*, 66.
10. Sontag, *Illness*, 102.
11. For example, Sheryl Stolberg, "Obama Pointedly Questioned by Students in India," *New York Times*, November 7, 2010 (extremism in Pakistan is "a cancer within the country"); Tamar Jacoby, "Lost in Juarez," *New York Times*, November 5, 2010 ("the deadly cancer of narcoviolence and corruption on the Mexican side"); "Debt Panel Head: Congress Must 'Face Up' to Issue," *New York Times*, November 15, 2010 ("The debt we are building up is like a cancer").
12. For example, American Cancer Society, "Questionable Cancer Practices in Mexico." Retrieved September 20, 2010, from www.cancer.org/Treatment/TreatmentsandSideEffects/ComplementaryandAlternativeMedicine/PharmacologicalandBiologicalTreatment/Index
13. "Fear: The Gap between American Actions and Attitudes on Cancer," *NCI Bulletin*, March 9, 2004. Retrieved September 2, 2010, from http://www.c-changetogether.org
14. Peggy Eastman, "Survey: About Half of Americans Unaware of Obesity's Link to Cancer," *Oncology Times*, December 25, 2009. A 2006 survey found

that cancer was the most feared disease among adults generally, although among people over age 55, Alzheimer's disease was the most frightening. "Older Americans Fear Alzheimer's the Most, While Most Adults Fear Cancer." Retrieved September 2, 2010, from http://seniorjournal.com/ NEWS/Alzheimers/6–05-31-OlderAmericans.htm

15. National Cancer Institute, Health Information Trends Survey. Retrieved September 15, 2010, from http://hints.cancer.gov/questions/section1.jsp?secti on=Cancer+Perceptions+and+Knowledge

16. "Survey: Americans Fear Paying for Cancer Treatment as Much as Dying of the Disease," *Oncology Times*, August 10, 2009. Retrieved September 15, 2010, from http://www.oncology-times.com

17. Tara Parker-Pope, "Fear and Procrastination Delay Cancer Diagnoses," *New York Times*, May 14, 2008. Retrieved September 2, 2010, from http:// well.blogs.nytimes.com/2008/05/14/fear-and-procrastination-delay-cancer- diagnoses/

18. See Nathan S. Consedine, Carol Magai, Yulia S. Krivoshekova, et al., "Fear, Anxiety, Worry and Breast Cancer Screening: A Critical Review," *Cancer Epidemiology, Biomarkers & Prevention* 13 (2004): 501–10.

19. For example, full-body computed tomography (CT) cancer screening has become popular, despite its risks and lack of proven benefit for healthy individuals with no signs or symptoms of disease. See U.S. Food and Drug Administration, "Full-Body CT Scans–What You Need to Know." Retrieved September 20, 2010, http://www.fda.gov/Radiation-EmittingProducts/ RadiationEmittingProductsandProcedures/MedicalImaging/. See also Renee Twombly, "Full-Body CT Screening: Preventing or Producing Cancer?" *Journal of the National Cancer Institute* 96 (2004): 1650–51.

20. Frank, *At the Will*, 83.

21. Frank, *At the Will*, 92.

22. Frank, *At the Will*, 94.

23. National Institutes of Health, "Estimates of Funding for Various Research, Condition, and Disease Categories," Feb. 1, 2010. Retrieved September 22, 2010, from http://report.nih.gov/rcdc/categories/

24. Robert Farley, "More Money, but a Long Ways from Doubling," *Politifact*, February 26, 2009. Retrieved September 22, 2010, from http://www. politifact.com/truth-o-meter/promises/promise/84/double-federal-funding- for-cancer/

25. Joel Finkelstein, "Texas Prepares to Invest Billions in Cancer Research," *Journal of the National Cancer Institute* 100 (2008): 696–97.

26. See generally Rebecca Dresser, *When Science Offers Salvation: Patient Advocacy and Research Ethics* (New York: Oxford University Press, 2001).

27. As Patterson notes, critics have been raising this question for years. See Patterson, *Dread Disease*, 243.

CHAPTER 10

Caregivers, Patients, and Clinicians

John A. Robertson

Caregiving for any serious disease, especially in its late stages, is stressful and difficult. In this chapter, I consider my experiences as a caregiver during my wife, Carlota Smith's, illness. As I described in Chapter 3, Carlota was diagnosed in May, 2005, with stage four ovarian cancer. She and I had two more years together. During that time, Carlota and I lived through surgery, many rounds of chemotherapy, and the final weeks of her life. Although the experience of being a caregiver is different from that of the patient, much is shared. In the pages that follow, I refer often to "our" cancer, which is for me the natural way to put it.

The cancer world is replete with medical and psychological issues for patients, family caregivers, and the doctors and nurses treating them. Most of the issues are not unique to cancer or any of its myriad variations; they arise in many other illness settings. But cancer gives us a perch from which to reflect more generally on the struggles that patients and caregivers face on life's downward spiral.

The specific struggles I recount reflect my experiences with Carlota's gynecological oncologist and the community cancer center in Austin, Texas, where Carlota was treated. As a caregiver, I learned about the rules of the cancer treatment game—how doctors and the rest of the medical staff expect patients and caregivers to behave, and how difficult it can be to challenge those expectations. I learned about the need for diplomacy—caregiving often calls for delicate negotiation with doctors and with the patient you love. I learned to be strong when

I wanted to run away and hide, though sometimes I did have to escape for a while. And I learned about living with the terror of knowing that nothing could be done to postpone for very long the ultimate outcome.

Arthur Kleinman, a medical anthropologist and caregiver for his wife, who has Alzheimer's disease, describes caregiving as "a defining moral practice," a practice that "make[s] us, even as we experience our limits and failures, more human."[1] The caregiving experience did make me more human. It left me battered and bruised, and I still feel its effects as I write three years after Carlota's death. But it also left me thankful for the privilege of being with a woman who was much stronger than I in facing our terrible situation. I hope that it has left me better prepared to deal with the illness and debilitation that I, and the people I know and love, will face in the future.

THE WORLD OF CANCER TREATMENT

By the time it was diagnosed, Carlota's cancer had spread throughout her abdomen, and her long-term prognosis was not good. But there were several things her doctor could do to give her a few more years of life. After she was diagnosed, Carlota had two rounds of chemotherapy to shrink the fluid in her belly so that surgery could occur. She then had surgery to remove her ovaries and "debulk" (an ugly and objectifying term that I still detest) the remaining cancer in her body. Then she had twelve more rounds of chemotherapy. The goal of chemotherapy after debulking surgery is not cure, but remission. Carlota lived for two years, but never made it to remission.

During the many months of Carlota's treatment, she and I learned how the health care system socializes those it serves into certain roles. Clinicians control information and send direct and indirect messages to teach people how to respond as good patients and family caregivers. There is a rhythm and routine to it all: checking into the cancer center; having a blood test to make sure the patient is "healthy" enough to withstand that day's drugs; waiting for a treatment chair to become available; having the chemotherapy; and three or four hours later, being discharged. For us, discharge involved checking out, making appointments for the white and red blood cell monitoring that was part of every chemotherapy cycle, scheduling the next chemotherapy session, and exchanging a bit of chit-chat with the clerical staff we came to know.

Carlota and I developed our own strategies for coping with the demands of her treatment. I would take Carlota to the cancer center and stay with her until she was cleared for that day's chemotherapy. Then I would go to my office, then back to the center, often bringing her lunch. While I was gone, she read linguistic papers or dozed off in the chemotherapy chair. Unlike other patients, Carlota did not want company during the whole session. I did the best I could to respect her wishes. I must admit that I too was glad for some time on my own.

When I was with Carlota, I paid attention as best as I could to the drugs she was given, on guard for any mistakes in the treatment regimen. I also worried that Carlota would be disturbed by the loud televisions in the unit. In truth, Carlota wasn't particularly bothered by them; I was the one who hated the noise. I concealed my irritation, though, not wanting to interfere with the other patients' way of dealing with chemotherapy.[2] In this ordeal, the patients had to come first.

And then it would be time to take Carlota home. At that point, she would be tired, her face flushed from Taxol, one of the chemotherapy drugs. Sometimes she was agitated, too, a side effect of the steroid that is routinely given with chemotherapy to prevent allergic reactions. We thought the agitation was just one more thing we had to put up with and didn't complain about it. But later, when Carlota mentioned the problem to a doctor, the doctor removed the steroid from the treatment regimen, explaining that patients who complained about agitation could go without it. Knowing when to complain and what to complain about is an ongoing challenge for patients and caregivers.

After chemotherapy, we hurried to get home, battling the rush-hour traffic and sometimes arguing about small matters like where to pick up groceries. Our anxiety and tension came out in little tiffs about which store had the best cookies to offer our many visitors. Carlota always preferred the specialty stores, which required a longer detour. I longed for the peace and security of our house, so I always favored the most convenient store. Because I, Mr. Efficiency, was the driver, I had the ultimate power over whether we would go the extra miles. Sometimes I used this power to get my way. Even when chemotherapy went well, it was stressful for us both.

The next day, we would head back to the cancer center for a blood test, and then back again in ten days for a booster shot to counteract some of chemotherapy's side effects.[3] What was especially scary was the monthly monitoring of CA-125 levels, the marker that indicated whether Carlota was responding to treatment. We were compelled to become experts on the rating and prognostic indicator on which so much of our lives would turn. This, too, was part of the socialization process.

When she was diagnosed in May 2005, Carlota had a CA-125 level of six thousand, truly off the charts. Two cycles of chemotherapy, surgery, and more chemotherapy brought it down to five hundred and then two hundred. Remission—and freedom from drugs—would come when the score was thirty for two months in a row. But we never made it below ninety-two. At that point, the number always started to climb back up. In an ironic twist, the higher numbers signaled the slide down to Carlota's demise, a slide the doctor warned would happen sooner or later. And then, as poet C.K. Williams put it, "later became sooner."[4]

When it was clear that the first-line drug regimen was no longer working, we turned to second-line therapies, hoping that they would hold the Furies at bay. Of course they did not, but we kept trying, unwilling to abandon hope, with its "bright feathers and its singing in the night without asking anything in return."[5] Second-line therapy was thalidomide and another drug that I can't bear to go back through the records to identify. This treatment regimen was being studied in a clinical trial, and it seemed reasonable to give it a try. But Carlota reacted very badly to the thalidomide. We tried a third and then a fourth treatment regimen, and then stopped.

I cannot imagine that anyone enjoys cancer treatment, but patients and families are socialized to maintain a positive outlook. The cancer center had a "cheery" atmosphere. This was not Solzhenitsyn's dreary Cancer Ward, but a bright and colorful place in a new building with nice furniture. The people running the place were also upbeat. Being so overwhelmed by cancer myself and seeing patients further along in the trajectory than Carlota was, I wondered how the doctors, nurses, aides, clerks—indeed, everyone involved in the delivery of cancer care—coped with the brooding omnipresence of death.

I was struck by how positive everyone was, or tried to be. Most of them succeeded in this effort, especially the bubbly phlebotomist who would usually draw Carlota's blood before that day's chemotherapy. The oncologist managing Carlota's care was upbeat, as well. She was helping us to stay alive, and we counted on her to keep us going. When she finished examining Carlota, she would always give her a quick hug as we walked out the door, and Carlota and I headed for the chemotherapy suite. No doubt she was well-defended against the sadness that her patients and their families were feeling, for how else could she do her job so effectively? Of course, we only saw the doctor at the treatment center. Perhaps the cheerful mask came off when she was away from work. The doctor also seemed to shut down later, when Carlota stopped responding to the chemotherapy. At that point, she handed us off to an outpatient hospice program, and turned her attention to the patients who could still benefit from treatment.[6]

Like the other members of our cancer ethics group, I was especially impressed by the chemotherapy nurses. They had many patients to monitor and little time for conversation as they maneuvered to get what everyone hoped were life-sustaining drugs into their patients. I wondered why they hadn't chosen a less depressing area of nursing and was startled when one of the younger nurses told us how much she preferred oncology over her previous post at a dialysis center. She thought that cancer patients had more hope and were more active than the dialysis patients she had cared for earlier.

Everyone at the cancer center seemed too busy, and the doctors and other staff weren't always as attentive as we wanted them to be. The oncologist in charge of Carlota's treatment was usually very helpful, but every so often, she dropped the ball. I was furious once when she did not return an e-mail message. Besides facing the usual fatigue and frustrations of an oncology practice, she was under financial pressure to carry a heavy patient load. The cancer center was a partnership owned by the doctors. Carlota's oncologist told us that she had to pay out of pocket to hire a nurse practitioner to help with patient care.

MY LIFE AS A CAREGIVER

I stood by Carlota's side while she went through cancer treatment, and she rewarded me with a special title. Carlota called me her "most favorite Chilla." The term comes from Rudyard Kipling's *Kim*,[7] a book we had listened to during our drive home from Big Bend National Park a few months before the cancer hit. Kim, the title character, is a half-breed street urchin who takes care of an aged holy man looking for the waters that heal all ills. Kim becomes the holy man's "chilla," a term referring to the one who helps another in his search, finding him food and lodging for the night and guiding him along the way. I am deeply honored that Carlota came up with that title for me. Although I could not find the healing waters that she needed, I was there helping her at every step along the way.

It took some time for me to become Carlota's most favorite Chilla. Carlota wanted to maintain her independence. She refused to let me treat her as if she were helpless and needy, which was what I initially thought I should do to protect her. Sometimes I was too intrusive and obsessive, trying to control what was uncontrollable. Carlota would object, and I eventually learned to back off. In her chapter, "Autonomy and Persuasion," Rebecca Dresser describes a similar dynamic that arose when her partner Peter was trying to convince her to accept a feeding tube during her cancer treatment. In our group discussion, Leon Kass spoke of his difficulties in finding the right balance between encouraging his wife to have a positive attitude about her cancer treatment, and accepting her need to express the anxiety she was feeling. In my experience as caregiver, the most important negotiation was with Carlota and how she wanted to live her illness, an illness I also was living. Sometimes when I thought I was protecting her, I was in fact trying to protect myself.

Besides helping her through the ups and downs of chemotherapy, I was Carlota's advocate. I felt I had a duty to do all I could to ensure that she got the best available treatment. For example, after Carlota's surgery, I pushed for a second opinion at M. D. Anderson, the well-regarded cancer hospital in Houston. I consulted a gynecologist I knew through my medical ethics work, and he recommended that we see the chairman of M. D. Anderson's gynecological oncology department. But Carlota's oncologist was more comfortable with a younger doctor there, someone she knew and trusted, and we took her advice.

Although we were glad for the opportunity to get a second opinion, arranging the appointment was complicated. It took many phone calls to get the local cancer center staff to forward Carlota's medical records, scans, tumor samples, and other information the Houston staff had to have before scheduling an appointment. The process was quite stressful—it was just after Carlota's surgery, and I was on edge. Every patient and caregiver in our cancer ethics group encountered similar problems. As Patricia Marshall described it, there were times when we "wanted to scream" at the people who weren't doing their jobs properly. But we were also dependent on those people. When they made mistakes, they expected patience and forbearance. So, we learned how to respond. To get what we wanted, we had to be both assertive and polite.

On the day before our appointment at M. D. Anderson, Carlota and I flew to Houston. We were joined by Judy, a good friend. I was glad to have another person along to support Carlota as we listened to what would probably be more bad news about her condition. Judy would also tape the session, so that we could go over information we failed to absorb in the intensity of the moment. I was well prepared for that meeting, with detailed questions about technical matters like molecular staging and monoclonal antibodies. Impressed, the doctor said, "You have done your homework." But it turned out that the treatments I had read about weren't relevant to Carlota's situation. My attempts to be useful in this regard did not succeed, but it was important to know that I had done what I could.

The doctor at M. D. Anderson gave us no new reason for optimism, but did confirm that our treatment plan—multiple rounds of chemotherapy with Taxol and carboplatin—was sound. Because the doctor still hadn't received a report from the M. D. Anderson pathologist, she wanted us to come back the next day. This meant getting a room for an extra night and changing our flight plans. We were not happy about this, but as we left the office, the doctor endeared herself to Carlota by saying she "liked Carlota's glasses" and owned a pair of the same stylish frames.

We had a rough afternoon and night in Houston. The death sentence had been confirmed and there was no way out. We stayed at the Ronald McDonald house for cancer patients, another warm and colorful facility. Despite the upbeat environment, we were glum and depressed. I remember sitting with our friend and going over the tape recording of what we had heard.

The next day was a little better, however. We were thrilled when the consultant oncologist said that there might have been a mistake in the original pathology report done in Austin. Carlota's primary cancer might not be ovarian, but a form of uterine cancer. Although this would not improve the prognosis, there was more research being conducted on uterine cancer and a somewhat better outlook. It lifted us and gave us hope—one of our few joyous moments in the medical morass that was engulfing us.

In the end, nothing we learned from the second opinion changed Carlota's diagnosis or treatment. Yet, we did develop a good relationship with the doctor at M. D. Anderson. She was conscientious and responded quickly to the e-mail messages Carlota and I sent when we had questions about our Austin doctor's recommendations. She was especially helpful when we faced the decision to stop further chemotherapy and go into outpatient hospice care.

Another part of my role as Carlota's advocate was to check the Internet for clinical trials evaluating treatments for the type of cancer Carlota had. When she was diagnosed, I did an online search and found many ovarian cancer trials. But none that I found seemed appropriate for her condition. And, without medical expertise, I couldn't tell whether my impression was correct. Carlota's oncologist did suggest one trial, but it turned out not to be suitable for us. Travel to an out-of-state center for trial participation was out of the question, because Carlota wanted to stay at home in Austin and continue her teaching. As Rebecca Dresser notes in her chapter on clinical trials, study enrollment isn't a real option for many cancer patients.

My experience as a caregiver gave me a better understanding of why many patients with advanced cancer want to try experimental treatments. During the course of Carlota's treatment, an organization representing terminally ill patients filed a lawsuit challenging the U.S. Food and Drug Administration's restrictions on patients' access to early-phase investigational drugs. I wrote a short article backing the right of the patient to get untested chemotherapy drugs.[8] No doubt I was influenced by Carlota's situation. Even though I personally oppose what I see as overuse of questionable-benefit drugs at the end of life, I thought that patients should be free to try such drugs if their doctor agreed and a drug company was willing to supply them.

I worked hard to deserve my position as Carlota's "most favorite Chilla." Yet there were times when the demands were too much. One of those times was when the red cells in Carlota's blood unexpectedly plummeted and she needed a transfusion. I had gone out of town for the day, and Carlota had driven herself the cancer center for a routine blood test. When I returned from my trip in the early evening, I expected Carlota to be home. I realized something was wrong when I saw that her car was gone and found a message light blinking on the telephone. But my travel day had been stressful and I really needed a break. I decided to postpone listening to the message until after I had a brief walk and a bite to eat. I knew that any problem was unlikely to be major, and I was afraid that the message would change my schedule. I was going to take care of myself first.

Once I listened to the message, I learned that Carlota was in the hospital receiving a transfusion. I drove to the hospital at once. The transfusion was finished, but Carlota had developed hives. Her doctor, usually so good on technical details, had forgotten to order the drug (Benadryl) that prevents allergic reactions in patients receiving transfusions. Carlota was spotty, red, and, understandably, unhappy. She had been waiting for her doctor to order the proper drug so she could feel better. The order finally came, and a couple of hours later we were back home, an evening lost. I never told Carlota about my forty-five minute delay in getting to the hospital, but I don't feel guilty about putting myself first on this occasion.

STANDING BY AND STANDING WITH
AT THE END OF LIFE

By the late fall of 2006, my caregiving role began to change. The treatment phase was coming to a close, and I faced new and terrifying responsibilities. The new phase began when we learned that what had been a two-centimeter tumor on top of Carlota's right adrenal gland was now twelve centimeters and growing. In December, after briefly examining Carlota, her oncologist said, "Let's get it out and buy some time." She was optimistic that surgery might give us an additional year. She wasn't qualified to do the surgery, but thought a local expert on adrenal surgery would be able to do what was needed. She was not able to reach him then, so she asked us to arrange the appointment and promised that she would assist in the surgery.

Setting up the appointment turned out to be much more difficult than we thought it would be. This is one time when I thought Carlota's doctor let us down. She should have talked with the other surgeon about Carlota's situation before sending us to him. (I also blame myself for not asking her to consult him first, though I pushed as much as seemed possible in the circumstances.) When we called the expert's office, we learned that he was away on a two-week vacation. We would not be permitted to schedule an appointment until he returned and agreed to see us. It was getting close to Christmas, and we had planned a trip to New York for early January. We didn't know whether to cancel the trip. Finally, Carlota decided we should go to New York. We told family and friends we would have the surgery when we got back.

I am glad that we went to New York, for this would be our final trip together. We did all that we usually did there, seeing friends and going to the theater and art museums. As usual, Carlota had more energy than I did (I have a lung condition called sarcoidosis that reduces my stamina). When we got home, we were finally able to see the expert. After some informal conversation (it turned out that the surgeon lived in our neighborhood), he said he could not do the operation. It would not be simple to remove the adrenal tumor, and there were so many other tumors in the abdomen that he didn't think surgery would help us. He said there was another surgeon in town we could consult, but he didn't think that doctor would be willing to operate either. The handwriting on the wall was coming into focus.

We went back to Carlota's oncologist, who said she hadn't thought the surgery would be so complicated. She then described our remaining options. She said we could try more chemotherapy, but it would be a once-a-week regimen, rather than the three-week cycle we were used to. Chemotherapy might give us a few more months, but Carlota would feel sick much of that time. It would be hard for her to continue to teach and be as active as she had been. It was a bleak picture, but Carlota said, "Let's do the chemo." Her doctor repeated that it would not be easy, the benefit was likely to be slight, and Carlota's quality of life would be poor. The doctor added that she herself, as well as many other patients in Carlota's situation, might choose to do nothing. The wisdom of that course immediately became apparent to both Carlota and me.

When a surgeon doesn't want to operate and an oncologist doesn't want to administer chemotherapy, they are telling you something. We grasped the import of their message, a message I am grateful they conveyed. But it took a day or two for Carlota and me to get comfortable with it. And we never explicitly acknowledged that we were crossing the threshold to the terminal phase of the illness. It helped that the doctor at M. D. Anderson sent us an e-mail note confirming the local oncologist's prognosis and recommendation.

A day or so later, we had to confront a hard question: whether to sign up for hospice care to manage the pain, which was becoming a problem for the first time in the course of Carlota's illness. Her oncologist wrote a prescription for pain medication, but said that the hospice staff would do a better job with pain management. The "hospice" label was difficult for both of us to accept, though I accepted it more easily because I wanted Carlota to have the best possible treatment for her pain.

Going into the hospice program meant that doctors believed Carlota had at most six months to live. Since she was still functioning well, we tried to block out this dire prediction, wanting to believe that her life would go on much longer. A conversation with our friend Judy a few days later helped us to accept it. I remember seeing Judy to the door on that cold and starry January night. I broke into tears and said, "Carlota is going to die, and there is nothing that we can do to stop it." Judy hugged me and said that she was there for us, and she was. She was there when Carlota was dying and was the first to notice that Carlota was telling us good-bye. She also presided at Carlota's memorial service and has remained a close friend.

Somehow we managed those last months. The pain became worse. Every few days, I would apply a patch with a higher dose of fentanyl, a pain medication, to Carlota's skin. Carlota also went to a Chinese doctor each week for acupuncture, which left her relaxed and upbeat.

(Mandarin was one of Carlota's linguistic specialties, and this helped her create one of those relational bonds she was so good at making.) She would always return with a contented, tranquil look on her face, so different from the way she looked after chemotherapy. Her hair also grew back, and she was her usual elegant self.

But Carlota's stomach was swelling up again, this time with tumors rather than fluid. This frightened me, for it was a visible sign that the cancer was conquering her body. I could not bring myself to touch her stomach until her daughter Alison did so on one of her last visits. After that, I was able to touch it, too. In the meantime, Carlota refused to give in to her illness. She kept up her work, teaching, seeing students, and doing other academic tasks. A month before she died, she ran an international conference on literature and linguistics, another of her academic specialties. When her children visited for Mother's Day, Carlota wanted to celebrate with a walk in Pedernales State Park, a favorite spot of ours. A picture of me helping her down the steps still rips me apart, because she had become so bony and frail.

As Carlota became sicker, I struggled with a complicated set of emotions. I wanted to stay by her side, but desperately needed a break. Carlota seemed to understand this and urged me to get away for a few days. I had hardly traveled since her illness, but went to Phoenix one night in early May to see a baseball game with old friends. I also decided, with Carlota's approval, to attend a one-day professional meeting in Chicago. It was scheduled for May 21, Carlota's birthday. I planned to return that evening and join her at a birthday dinner that friends were giving.

When I left Sunday afternoon for the airport, Carlota was talking on the phone to an old friend. I was resentful that she would not interrupt the call to tell me goodbye, yet I was actually leaving for the airport earlier than I needed to. And, once the plane was airborne, I regretted my decision to go to the meeting.

As soon as I got to Chicago, I called Carlota, and we had a warm and loving conversation. But I was a wreck the next day, nervous and distracted. Fortunately, my flight arrived in Austin on time, and I made it to the birthday dinner. I could tell immediately that Carlota was not doing well and quickly took her home. She told me she had almost blacked out while driving home from her office at the height of rush hour. But she didn't want to admit how ill she was. She said she wanted to attend the Navajo Institute Summer Camp in New Mexico that July. I knew it was unlikely she would make it there, but said, "Of course, we will go."

The next morning, Carlota awoke in great pain. The hospice nurse said we should go to the inpatient hospice facility immediately, so that they could get the pain under control. We went, thinking it would be a temporary stay. A hospice nurse gave Carlota what the nurse and I referred to as "sublingual" morphine. We had a lighthearted moment when Carlota, who hated technical jargon, insisted on calling it morphine "under the tongue."

We were glad for the pain medication, but weren't completely happy with our introduction to the hospice facility. We had expected the staff to be kind and competent, which they were for the most part. But that first day, we had to put up with an officious and unpleasant Scottish nurse. And we didn't like having to listen to a music therapy student play "Danny Boy" on the harp. Things got better when two very close friends came to be with us. One friend stayed with Carlota that night so that I could go home and try to sleep.

I spent the next morning with Carlota. In the afternoon, I went to my office for a brief respite and then returned to the hospice. Two events stand out. Carlota was able to leave her bed to have a shower and her hair washed. A small victory, but it made us both feel better. Once she was back in bed, she pointed to an air-conditioning vent high on the south wall and said it was like the vent in a hospital room she had occupied after surgery. Confused, I said I thought the hospital vent was on the other side of the room. I didn't understand that she meant something much more significant. In pointing upward, she was telling me that she would soon be going into the air.[9] In a similar vein, she told our friend Judy that "she was following the green road and would be leaving tomorrow." I regret that I missed these signals that Carlota was preparing to die.

By now, Carlota was resting a lot. I couldn't sit still and wandered around outside. In the early evening, while I was chatting with a chaplain, a nurse came and told me to contact Carlota's children—she was going downhill. I made the awful phone call, and they both managed to get there from the East Coast before Carlota died. No memory is more poignant to me than seeing Carlota's daughter Alison sitting on the bed as Carlota smiled and stroked her hair. Carlota's son Joel arrived a few hours later, when Carlota was still breathing, but unconscious. At about six o'clock, her breathing slowed and, at 6:50, a nurse pronounced her dead.

Consistent with Carlota's general unwillingness to speak openly about the fact that she was dying, we had not discussed funeral arrangements. But long before her illness, Carlota had told me that she wanted to be cremated. I called a funeral home and waited for someone to come and get her cold body. I told Carlota's children to go home and rest, that I would take care of the formalities. I thought that they needed a break, and I wanted some time alone with Carlota's stiffening body. It was Memorial Day weekend, the same time of year that we had learned of Carlota's diagnosis and started this journey to the bottom. A thunderstorm had blown in, and the man from the funeral home was delayed. Once he arrived, I signed the necessary papers and watched as he loaded Carlota into a bag, which he put on a gurney. He pushed the gurney out of the room and disappeared into the late spring rain.

The day after Carlota died, I was utterly exhausted. In the moments I was alone, I howled in grief. But I had to keep going, for there were many things I needed to do. I called friends and family and helped Carlota's daughter write an obituary. We decided to hold a memorial service the following weekend, rather than wait until the fall. But we were upset to discover that we would not get Carlota's ashes in time for the service. The cremation had been delayed due to the Memorial Day back-up in the medical examiner's office.

That day, I also sent Carlota's oncologist, whom we had not seen for a few months, an e-mail message saying, "This magnificent woman has died." I yearned for a response—a few words saying how sorry she was—but got none. I called her office the next day and told the nurse that I had sent the doctor an e-mail and was hoping to have a response. I never got one. Weeks later, the cancer center sent a large card with fulsome notes from the nurses and staff who had come to know Carlota. There was also a very brief condolence from the doctor. Given our relationship, this seemed insufficient, but perhaps I was unreasonable in expecting more from an oncologist whose patients were always dying and who had many living patients to look after.

Arranging the memorial service took all of my remaining energy. It turned out that some very close friends were unable to attend. They had good reasons for missing the service, but I still resented their absence. I wanted everyone to mark the occasion, to acknowledge the gravity of what had occurred. I decided to speak at the service and struggled to come up with the right remarks. In a moving tribute to Carlota, the University of Texas president ordered the flags outside a landmark campus building flown at half mast. They snapped in the strong wind as Carlota's son Joel took pictures of them. I was able to hold it together at the memorial service, ending my appreciation of Carlota with a poem prefiguring death, a poem she had chosen to read at our last poetry group.[10]

The next night, our families and out-of-town friends departed. I was left alone with my grief and heavy heart at the loss of Carlota, that magnificent woman I was so blessed to have as my wife.

When death occurs, the caregiver becomes a grieving spouse. For me, grief has been a relentless and punishing experience, one that has consumed my life for three years. Yes, tincture of time has helped make it better, but the grief is still there. I have not been able to have pictures of Carlota visible in the house, because it is so painful to look at her and feel her absence. But I sense that one day I will be able to focus on the great gifts I received during my sixteen years with Carlota. A writer who went through a similar ordeal put into words my own state of mind:

> This grief is not to be dismissed by some attempted appeal to reason. Not now. Not ever. But it may help from time to time to look at the underside of this pain—as one lifts a leaf to look at the silvery underside—and note what riches we have had in the life of this one whose death we mourn.
>
> Sometime down the road—and when that will be is as variable as the people who mourn—the grief will be on the underside and the sense of blessingand gratitude will be the bright surface, luminous and green.[11]

THE BURDENS OF CAREGIVING

Caring for a loved one with terminal cancer inflicts physical and psychological damage. Studies have shown that caregivers experience psychological difficulties equal to or even greater than those of patients.[12] Yet, when I was a caregiver, clinicians often expected me to act as their medical assistant. Not many of them seemed aware that my emotional state was closer to that of a patient than a detached professional. Nor did they seem aware of the caregiver's struggles, including conflicts with the patient, doctors, and family members. So, I agree with the experts who say that caregiver distress should receive more attention than it usually receives. I also agree that "[p]revention of the family caregiver's burden should become an integral part of good palliative care . . . for the terminally ill."[13]

My full-throated account of Carlota's illness conveys how distressing the experience was for me. Although we did not have family nearby, we had close friends, a therapist, a good medical team, good insurance coverage, and many more sources of support to help us through.

I cannot conceive of how families without financial means or flexible work schedules cope with the crisis of terminal cancer.

Despite having all of these advantages, Carlota's illness and the grief that has followed it has been the most stressful experience of my life. During this period, I lost over thirty pounds and had a minor car accident. I was distracted and unfocused, and I felt hopeless. It's hard for me to imagine how Patricia Marshall managed to function as a caregiver in circumstances even worse than the ones I experienced. Patty was still dealing with her own breast cancer when her husband, Larry, was diagnosed with the rapidly progressing cancer that ended his life in a matter of weeks. Patty told us she had no time to think about her burdens, and no choice but to act: "It was like we were on a train rushing into a stone wall," she said.

One of the most difficult aspects of my own situation was Carlota's refusal to talk openly about the death she was facing. Her way of moving forward was to concentrate on her work and the concrete medical activities that took over much of our lives. I once made a clumsy attempt to talk to her about the "elephant in the room," but she quickly rebuffed me, saying, "I don't want to talk about it." Carlota hardly ever grumbled about her plight or even mentioned her deepest feelings and fears to me. I later learned she had expressed them in e-mail messages to her friends. She also put her thoughts about dying into a diary, which she forbade me to read after her death.[14]

Carlota revealed her true emotions to me just once. In the second year of her illness, she lifted the veil and said to me, "If only I could feel good again." We both knew that this would probably happen rarely, if at all. The remark about "wanting to feel good again" showed me how miserable she really was. She played her cards close to the chest, but this was a slip.

Although I sometimes wanted to confront our situation more directly, I see now that Carlota's reserve was a *mitzvah*, a gift to me. She realized that talking and sharing would have made it more difficult for both of us. And she was right. Neither one of us wanted the cancer to be center stage, with the klieg lights of fear and panic shining in the darkness. We wished the cancer would fade away and disappear, but knew that it wouldn't. So, we had to deny and distance. We pretended that it wasn't there, though we could never really forget it. As Carlota's closest friend put it, "She lived the cancer on two levels: she knew she was going to die and then wanted to get on with her life as a linguist and mother and spouse."

Besides sadness, I have some guilt about my behavior toward the end of Carlota's life. I realize that I was responding to my need to withdraw from what was an excruciatingly painful experience. I think Carlota understood this, for she encouraged me to go on the two trips I made soon before her death. As Rebecca pointed out in our cancer group discussions, patients feel guilty for imposing responsibilities, as well as sadness, on their caregivers. Just as I wanted to help Carlota with her burdens, she wanted to help me with mine.

FINDING GOOD IN CANCER CAREGIVING

Not everything about being a caregiver was awful. Carlota and I were never closer than we were during the final two years of her life. And being a caregiver changed the way I look at the world. My experiences are consistent with recent studies showing that "both patients and their families can find benefit in the challenges associated with cancer."[15] These studies point to the phenomenon of personal growth or change after an encounter with a challenging or traumatic life experience. Most studies focus on the experiences of cancer survivors, but researchers have also looked at how family members may benefit from the challenge of caring for close relatives with cancer. They say that family caregivers may experience positive changes in five domains: new possibilities, relating to others, personal strength, appreciation of life, and spiritual change. Benefits like this do not "negate the adverse impact of the event," but are an important dimension in understanding how family members cope with their loss.[16]

After three years of grieving for Carlota and two years of living with her cancer and her struggles, I am still working to find the good in this experience. At this point, I at least know that I will be able to go on—a serious question for me in the months after her death. But will I go on imbued with Carlota and her gifts of modesty and generosity? I am trying to be more patient, open, and sensitive to others, as well as less insecure than I was before (after all, what could be worse than losing Carlota?). I am much better now at reaching out to people who face cancer or have lost a loved one.

A friend says that I have changed for the better, as a legacy from Carlota. I certainly hope I am better in some way. I would like to have something to show for all that wailing and gnashing of teeth. To go on blithely as before would be a worse loss, truly "an expense of spirit in a waste of shame."[17] Carlota gave me and everyone who knew her a lesson in how to live while dying. I have more studying to do before I'll be ready for my own time. When it comes, I hope I'm able to show just a bit of the grace and optimism she kept to the end.

Notes

1. Arthur Kleinman, "Caregiving: The Odyssey of Becoming More Human," *Lancet* 373 (2009): 292–93.
2. I am trying to follow Carlota's example and be less fussy about noise, but must admit I still cannot bear a blaring television.
3. Like many cancer patients, Carlota and other patients in our cancer ethics group were given injections of drugs designed to restore the red blood cells that chemotherapy destroys. In 2007, evidence emerged that the standard drug dose for cancer patients was too high, inducing strokes or cancer itself. Andrew Pollack, "Panel Seeks New Limits on Anemia Drugs," *New York Times*, March 14, 2008. Our group wondered whether financial interests accounted for the failure to study the drugs more carefully before they were used in so many patients.
4. C. K. Williams, "When," in *Selected Poems* (New York: Farrar, Straus, and Giroux, 1994), 193–94.
5. Emily Dickinson, "Hope Is the Thing with Feathers," in *The Laurel Poetry Series. Emily Dickinson* (New York: Dell, 1960), 35.
6. Arthur Frank's insights are relevant here:

   > Medical staff . . . are trapped by a belief that unless they can do something to reduce the bodily suffering, they have failed as professionals. Continuing suffering threatens them, so they deny it exists. What they cannot treat, the patient is not allowed to experience. Physicians and nurses often forget that when treatment runs out, there can still be care. Simply recognizing suffering for what it is, regardless of whether it can be treated, is care. Professionals can and do care, but when they do they are acting a bit unprofessional. . . . Sadly, the standard of what is "professional" often denies the opportunity of care.

   At the Will of the Body: Reflections on Illness (New York: Mariner Books, 2002), 101–102.
7. Rudyard Kipling, *Kim* (New York: Oxford University Press, 1987).
8. John Robertson, "Controversial Medical Treatment and the Right to Health Care," 36 *Hastings Center Report*, November-December, 2006, at 15–20. In 2007, a federal appellate court held that the U.S. Constitution does not give patients a right of access to experimental drugs. *Abigail Alliance for Better Access to Developmental Drugs v. Von Eschenbach*, 495 F.3d 695 (D. C. Cir. 2007).
9. I found this out only after Carlota died, when my therapist and a few others told me such actions were a characteristic sign of knowledge of approaching death.

10. The poem was George Meredith's "Dirge in Woods," with its haunting lines about pine trees "dropping their dead" needles, while, "Overhead, overhead/ Rushes life in a race/As the clouds the clouds chase/And we go/And we drop like the fruits of the tree/Even we/Even so." George Meredith, "Dirge in the Woods," in *Poems* (New York: Scribner, 1918), 350.

11. Martha Whitmore Hickman, *Healing after Loss: Daily Meditations for Working Through Grief* (New York: Harper Collins, 2002), May 26.

12. Serge Dumont, et al., "Caring for a Loved One with Advanced Cancer: Determinants of Psychological Distress in Family Caregivers," *Journal of Palliative Medicine* 9 (2006): 912–20.

13. Dumont, et al., "Caring," 917–18.

14. I found the diary after her death, opened it, saw something painful that she had written about me, and quickly closed it. I knew the diary would be toxic and, with the help of Norman Fost's wise counsel, managed to destroy it without looking at any other entries.

15. Youngmee Kim, Richard Schulz, and Charles S. Carver, "Benefit Finding in the Cancer Caregiving Experience," *Psychosomatic Medicine* 69 (2007): 283–91.

16. Kim, et al., "Benefit Finding," 286.

17. William Shakespeare, "Sonnet 129," in *The Sonnets* (New York: Penguin Books, 1964), 129.

CHAPTER II

Cancer Interactions

Caring Well and Caring Badly

Rebecca Dresser and Patricia A. Marshall

> *There ought to be behind the door of every happy, contented man*
> *someone standing with a hammer continually reminding him*
> *with a tap that there are unhappy people; that however happy he may*
> *be, life will show him her laws sooner or later, trouble will come for*
> *him—disease, poverty, losses, and no one will see or hear, just as now*
> *he neither sees nor hears others.*[1]

Cancer brings immersion in the medical system and removal from ordinary life. But connections to the outside world remain. Most patients spend more time out of hospitals and treatment centers than in them. Patients are at home, where relatives and friends can call or drop by. The lucky ones are able to leave the house for walks around the neighborhood, shopping, movies, and brief trips to the office. During these times, cancer patients interact with neighbors, co-workers, and strangers, and those interactions are changed by the presence of cancer.

The changes go in two directions. When we were cancer patients, and Patty's husband, Larry Heinrich, had terminal cancer, our relatives, friends, and acquaintances were more solicitous than we could ever have imagined in our pre-cancer lives. They lifted us up, reminding us of why it is good to be alive. But people let us down, too. We saw for ourselves the discomfort and insensitivity that a cancer diagnosis can provoke. We still remember both the wonderful and the disturbing reactions we witnessed during our cancer ordeals.

People dealing with cancer are needy and vulnerable. Many are frightened and on guard, hypersensitive to what others say and do. They feel immense gratitude when concern and caring seem genuine. But thoughtless remarks and callous behavior do more than their usual damage. Everyday interactions have an enormous impact on people facing cancer. In this chapter, we describe what personal experience taught us about helpful and harmful cancer interactions.

CASES IN POINT

After Rebecca was diagnosed with cancer, she went to the mall to buy comfortable clothes to wear during treatment. She is a planner, and the excursion was one way to gear up for the task ahead. She had lost weight, and her old clothes didn't fit anymore. She knew she would be stuck at home much of the time and was bound and determined not to lie around in pajamas all day. She would make every effort to get cleaned up and dressed every morning, no matter how wretched she felt. Shopping was also a pleasant distraction from the medical appointments and other depressing activities that come with a cancer diagnosis.

While engaged in her cancer shopping, Rebecca ran into someone she recognized. This was not someone she knew well, but etiquette required at least a brief chat. They made small talk, and he eventually asked why she was at the mall that day. She hesitated, but then answered truthfully. For a moment, he looked nervous, at a loss for words. Then he began talking about the medical difficulties his elderly parents were having, and his own struggles to assist them. She dutifully expressed sympathy. After that, he proceeded to tell her how much he was looking forward to his upcoming semester on leave in California. Now it was her turn to be at a loss for words. Why was he being so cruel? While she was suffering through treatment, he would be having the time of his life. She did not know how to respond to his insensitivity.

After Patty was diagnosed with breast cancer, she had a lumpectomy and then chemotherapy. One day, at the medical center, Patty struck up a conversation with another woman waiting in the hallway. Not surprisingly, they spoke of medical matters. Patty described her diagnosis and the treatment regimen she had chosen. She was stunned by the woman's response. The woman told Patty that she had been wrong to choose a lumpectomy. If Patty wanted to maximize her survival odds, she should have had a mastectomy instead.

Patty was standing during this conversation, leaning against the wall and feeling sick. She had severe fatigue and other bad side effects from the chemotherapy drugs she was receiving. She wasn't in the mood for a long discussion, but tried to explain that clinical trials had shown that lumpectomy was an effective treatment for tumors of the size and type that she had. But she wondered why she needed to defend her decision to someone she barely knew.

A few minutes later, it became clear that this woman was responding to her own medical worries. She said she was afraid she had one of the genes associated with high rates of breast cancer and was considering a mastectomy as a way to reduce her risk. Patty was tempted to tell the woman that a mastectomy couldn't completely protect her from cancer. But she held back, because she knew that this woman's decision was really none of her business. Although the woman felt free to second-guess Patty's medical decision-making, Patty wasn't about to do the same to her.

When Patty's husband Larry was dying from a rare and very aggressive form of lymphoma, he told her he hoped to die at home. He wanted to spend his last days on the sun porch of their old house, an embracing and comfortable room filled with books and light from windows on three sides. Patty rented a hospital bed and assembled the paraphernalia of the sickroom: a side table for medicines and water, a basin for washing adult diapers, and a "potty" in the corner. She put a chair by the bed for the friends and neighbors who stopped by to visit. Their golden retriever pup, Mr. Bentley, quietly observed the scene from his position under the bed. When Larry looked out the window, he could see the beautiful Japanese maple that their son and brother-in-law had planted for him.

This description suggests a peaceful place of dying, but the reality was far from tranquil. Larry's pain was horrific. The medications to control it weren't completely effective, and the steroid he was on made him paranoid and delusional. He often grimaced in pain, tossing and turning, not able to rest. He lost a lot of weight and looked terrible. Nevertheless, several of his visitors said to Patty, "Oh, he's looking so good!" or "Larry is really looking better!"

To Patty, the comments were bizarre. When she heard them, she wanted to reply, "Are you blind?" But she would murmur something socially appropriate, trying to help the person feel comfortable in the face of death's coming. Every so often, though, the disconnect between what was said and the reality of Larry's dying was too much to bear. When a visiting hospice nurse was making cheery comments about Larry's health, Patty finally said, "What are you saying? He's dying now! He does not look good! He is leaving us! His body is filled with cancer!"

CANCER'S "EXCUSE ME?" MOMENTS

These are a few examples of the clumsy and upsetting behavior we encountered when we were dealing with cancer. It wasn't unusual for people to bring up their own health worries, and sometimes it seemed as though they were trying to compete with us. We also heard a lot about upcoming travel plans, successes at work, and other highlights of the nice lives they were living. Someone even had the nerve to tell one of us that having cancer would be "a good challenge, a good learning experience." And, when Patty's husband Larry was dying, more than one person assured her that he would get better. Refusing to accept reality, they pretended that a miracle would halt cancer's relentless assault on his body.

People dealing with cancer often hear these kinds of remarks. A website called cancerchicks.com collects examples from across the country. Displayed under the heading, "Excuse Me?" they are introduced with the following questions:

Can you believe what some people are saying to you?
Can educated medical professionals really be that insensitive?
Can your normally intelligent family and friends really be that stupid?
Can't anyone see how very fragile you are right now?[2]

Our own "excuse me?" moments left us feeling isolated and lonely. They emphasized the disparity between the lives we were living and the ones ordinary people were privileged to have. Some of what we heard made us angry and defensive, too. We expected people to recognize the magnitude of what we were facing, not act as though it was business as usual. We don't think anyone meant to hurt us, but some of them, including a few close friends, did inflict injury. It seemed to us wrong that they hadn't bothered to think about the impact of their words.

Then there were the people who responded to our cancer with silence. Some of the people we expected to be present in our stories never made an appearance. They never said they were sorry to hear of our illness, never tried to be helpful. They were too intimidated—in our view, too cowardly—to do anything at all. Perhaps they were too focused on their own discomfort to recognize the crises we were facing.

We aren't psychologists, but we think we know why people acted this way. Our best guess is that they were trying to distance themselves from a situation that scared them. Their reactions were not about us, but about them. In us, they saw the essential vulnerability of being human. We were vivid reminders of the illness, loss, and mortality they would face in the future. We had once been full of vitality and energy and health. If cancer could happen to us, then surely it could happen to them. So, they avoided, denied, glossed over the reality of what we were confronting.

We suspect that ignorance also contributed to the unintended cruelty. In this culture, no one teaches us how to respond to people facing their own or a loved one's mortality. Despite all the public talk about living wills and death with dignity, few people are equipped to engage with someone confronting life-threatening illness. In a culture that has cast aside religious and other rituals associated with illness and death, many of us don't know how to respond to these misfortunes in real life.

Years after our cancer experiences, we have a better understanding of why people behave badly toward individuals dealing with cancer. We're even able to laugh about some of the idiotic remarks we heard—remarks like, "Deodorant must have caused your cancer," and "Maybe it was the unnatural additives they put in our food," and "Why did this happen to you?" But earlier, when cancer was the central focus of our lives, thoughtless words and actions caused unnecessary wounds. People ought to know and do better.

MISSTEPS AND MISDEEDS

Before cancer, members of our cancer ethics group were unaware of the range of reactions people have when someone they know is seriously ill. We've given some examples of the reactions we encountered, but have more tales to tell.

Certain individuals seemed to consider themselves cancer authorities, despite their lack of medical expertise or personal cancer experience.

Like the woman in Patty's story, some people thought they knew which treatment would be best for us. Others recommended certain doctors or urged us to travel to high-profile cancer centers far from our homes. People had lots of advice on lifestyle choices, too. Several members of our cancer ethics group received this sort of advice, but Patty's description was the most entertaining:

> I cannot tell you how much advice I was given. With my breast cancer, people were telling me, "Eat yogurt, do yoga, go on a macrobiotic diet, meditate, and oh by the way, relax, it's so important to relax!" The bluntness of some of the advice was startling. Also, if I heard one more person tell me to do yoga, I was just going to die. I listened to the advice, and here's what would go through my mind: "I can't take any more advice!" That is how it felt. There was a sense of being burdened, burdened by other people's stuff.

The advice-givers may have meant well, but much of their advice was unwelcome. A lot of it seemed silly to us—we are people who believe in evidence-based medicine. There was no way we were going to try an unproven remedy someone had found on the Internet. Some of the advice was presumptuous, too. What gave these people the right to tell us what we ought to do? What made them think they were qualified to decide what was best for us? And why did we have to put up with their need to take control of the situation?

We also resented the notion that there were simple remedies for our cancer and the treatment side effects we were experiencing. It seemed to diminish the gravity of our situation. Yogurt is certainly healthy to eat, and doing yoga helps some cancer patients handle anxiety and stress. But did people really think that our cancer would be affected by things like yoga and yogurt? Furthermore, we weren't interested in joining a yoga class while we were going through treatment; we were juggling too many appointments and obligations as it was. We held our tongues and listened politely, but found these exchanges extremely annoying.

When we were with friends and relatives, we felt duty-bound to put on a brave face, too. People would comment on our strength and courage, as if we were special. They would evoke the "warrior" image and say things like, "You're so strong—I know you'll be able to fight this battle and win!" Arthur Frank put it well in *At the Will of the Body*: "Everyone around the ill person becomes committed to the idea that recovery is the only outcome worth thinking about. No matter what the actual odds, an attitude of 'You're going to be fine' dominates the sickroom. Everyone works to sustain it."[3] Much of the time, the encouragement felt good. But no one really knew whether we would make it, and we weren't always in the mood to act as though they did. As Art observes, it takes work to maintain the optimistic front that helps others deal with your cancer.

In a similar vein, people often told us how good we looked. Some of them were telling white lies, for we knew we often looked pretty bad. The ones telling the truth must have thought cancer would make us look even worse than we did. Whatever their motivation, it was hard to know how to respond. Sometimes we would play along, sometimes we would argue the point. The worst moments were when people told Patty that Larry was looking better. He was dying, and she had to accept that. Making a sugar-coated comment about his appearance was no help at all.

Although there were times we couldn't abide the insistent optimism, we didn't like it when people were too grim, either. Some people acted as though we were already on our deathbeds. It was clear that they cared, but talking with them was a definite downer. Once, when Rebecca was telling someone how cancer had changed her priorities, the other person remarked, "You must be happy just to be able to draw your next breath." This sort of gloom and doom was the last thing we needed. We thought about worst-case scenarios enough on our own; we didn't need to hear about them from other people.

Cancer also reduced our tolerance for the superficial. We had trouble talking with people about the problems of everyday life. When people complained about their struggles to lose weight or keep up with their work, it was difficult to be sympathetic. Many of their concerns seemed petty, even though we recognized that we had once been absorbed in similar trifles. Their whining got on our nerves—they had no idea what it meant to have problems like the ones we were facing. We had to restrain ourselves from telling them how lucky they were to have such trivial worries.

It became more difficult to observe certain social conventions, as well. In ordinary life, "How are you?" is a polite greeting, not an invitation to self-revelation. But the standard answer, "Fine," seemed unacceptably phony when we were dealing with cancer. Early on, we gave everyone an authentic response, which was some variation of "not well." Some people were genuinely interested and could handle our honesty. Yet, we also learned that, as John Robertson put it, "So many times it's a mistake to say, 'Well, you know, I'm doing terrible.' They don't want to hear that, even though they say, 'No, *tell* me, how are you doing?'" So we developed brief responses that seemed less deceptive than "I'm fine." We would say, "All things considered, fine," or "I'm managing," or "As well as can be expected." Leon Kass came up with the best one, a traditional Polish reply: "Let's say, fine."

Certain institutional efforts to help cancer patients also fell flat. Some of the volunteers at the cancer center didn't have much to offer. They couldn't answer most of our questions and didn't have much to say other than, "How are you?" and "Could I bring you a snack?" We were irritated when they interrupted our reading or tried to interest us in art activities while we waited for chemotherapy. This was serious stuff, not a kindergarten class! Even the hospice volunteers sometimes got it wrong, as John and his wife Carlota Smith discovered when a music therapy student came to Carlota's hospice room to play "Danny Boy" on the harp. Neither Carlota nor John found this relaxing; indeed, it seemed to them an invasion of their privacy.

Rebecca witnessed one particularly misguided volunteer event. This was "Colon Cancer Awareness Day," celebrated in the chemotherapy center waiting room. Smiling people passed out information on colon cancer and samples of the types of food people should eat to avoid the disease. There were balloons, loud music, and cheerful speeches. Everyone seemed happy except the people who had come to the center for chemotherapy. A crowded and noisy room smelling of food was just about the worst place for a group of weary and nauseated cancer patients. We are all for teaching people about healthy lifestyles, but why do it in a place that is off-limits to the general public, a place full of very sick people in need of peace and quiet? A program that was undoubtedly intended to boost patients' morale ended up having the opposite effect.

It's not that we want to banish volunteers from the hospital and treatment center. Indeed, the work of volunteers provides considerable comfort to many patients and families. Bedside chats, art projects, and music therapy offer welcome breaks to children and adults seeking company, conversation, and the calming influence of music. And there was one volunteer effort that Patty really appreciated. During her chemotherapy treatments and Larry's hospitalizations, volunteers sometimes brought therapy dogs to the medical center. Watching the dogs, patients, and families enjoy each other was a wonderful distraction, a warm touch in a sterile and institutional environment. But Patty is a dog-lover, and it's possible that some patients didn't welcome these nonhuman visitors. Our point is that patients and their families may sometimes find volunteer activities intrusive. The best volunteer programs will seek advice from patients on how to be helpful, and will make it easy for patients to opt out if that's what they prefer.

UNEXPECTED OBLIGATIONS

Members of our cancer ethics group discovered that cancer creates new social responsibilities. For example, after we were diagnosed, we had to break the bad news to others. We had only begun to absorb what the doctors had told us, but it seemed vital to alert our families and close friends. In Chapter 3, John Robertson writes about the challenges doctors face in breaking bad news, but the task is even harder for patients. Most of the people in our group were unprepared for it. And though having cancer wasn't something we could control, we felt guilty imposing our news on the people we loved. It was especially hard when our loved ones sought assurances that we would get better, that the situation wasn't as bad as it sounded.

The day that Larry was diagnosed, he and Patty went home, poured themselves some whiskey, and spent many hours on the phone with children, brothers and sisters, and other loved ones. Although it was stressful and sad, they were rewarded with affirmation and love. Rebecca worried most about how to break the news to her elderly mother, who has dementia. Rebecca's mother lost her husband to cancer when he was thirty-nine, and because of the dementia, her mother has trouble remembering new information. To Rebecca's mother, cancer is a death sentence. What is the best way to tell someone so physically and mentally fragile that her child is facing the same disease that made her a widow?

Eventually we had to tell our co-workers, too, for someone would have to fill in for us during the worst phases of cancer treatment. It was awkward sharing such personal information with people we didn't know all that well. And then we had to tell our students. We knew that our news would be a shock to them, for not many had witnessed life-threatening illness close up. So, we had to think carefully about what to say and how to say it. We tried to be gentle and reassuring, and we tried not to cry when we saw some of them tear up while we were speaking.

Once we started telling people about our cancer, they passed on our news to others. People began writing and calling to express their concern. We were amazed and gratified by the number of messages we received. The hard part was responding to all of them. We wanted to thank everyone and answer all their questions, but we didn't always have the energy to get back to them. For Patty, going through treatment, caring for Larry, and grieving his loss left her so exhausted that she would "run out of words" for the well-wishers. Norman Fost came up with a good solution: sending mass e-mail bulletins to friends and colleagues. But the rest of us weren't organized enough to do that. We probably failed to get in touch with everyone who wrote or called, and in turn caused some hurt feelings.

Mass e-mails don't do the trick when people want to make personal contact, and we discovered that many people wanted that contact. They wanted to talk on the phone or come by the house for a visit. We too were eager for contact, and calls and visits were wonderful at the right time. Yet, there were times we couldn't manage conversation, and begged off, hoping they would understand. We tried to be gracious about it, but may have offended some people.

We were inundated with offers of help, too. This was truly heart-warming, but then we had to figure out something for people to do. At times, it was a real chore to come up with a task that would make them feel useful. We worried that people would feel rejected if we didn't give them an assignment. Again, Norm came up with a systematic approach. He gave people specific instructions on what would be helpful: walking the dog, grocery shopping, and so forth. Neither of us was capable of such an orderly response, though. During much of her treatment, Rebecca was too debilitated to cope with much of anything; for a few weeks, she had no voice at all due to the side effects of radiation treatment. When her husband Larry was sick, Patty was too overwhelmed to manage the offers of help. Each day presented a new crisis, and Larry needed round-the-clock care at the end of his life. She ended up asking some of their helpers to decide what the others could do to lessen her burden.

We realize there are traces of arrogance and narcissism in our reactions to cancer encounters. We freely admit it—we were more self-centered than usual when we had cancer. We wanted attention, and we wanted control over the conversation. We wanted to talk about what was on our minds. We wanted the freedom to decide whether to talk about cancer, or about something entirely different. And we didn't want to be burdened with worries about minding our manners.

We wanted people to give us respect, too. We were being tested in ways that few of them could imagine. We knew much more about facing serious illness than they did. Yet, some people seemed to look down on us. They spoke to us with pity, with heads lowered and faces full of sorrow. But their pity didn't make us feel better, and we didn't want to be seen as victims. To us, their reaction was demeaning, rather than comforting.

When we were dealing with cancer, we were not on our best behavior. Life was too hard and too complicated for us to observe all the rules of etiquette, much less keep up with everyone else's needs. We hope people realize that cancer can have this effect, and will forgive patients and caregivers for the occasional discourtesy.

GIFTS AND BLESSINGS

So far, we have concentrated on bad behavior, because we feel an urgent need to tell people about the unintended damage they can inflict. But we have things to say about good behavior, too. Plenty of people offered genuine comfort while we were coping with cancer, and some of them offered much more than that. We were blessed to know a few members of a select group novelist Elisa Albert describes as "people, rare, rare people, who can stare into the lonely, mysterious everlasting right alongside you, who can hold your hand, and who do not flinch from any part of whatever horrendous ordeal is at hand."[4]

Everyone in our cancer group was astonished and delighted at the support we received. Many people were magnificent, sending e-mail messages, cards, and other expressions of concern. Friends teamed up to bring flowers and food each week. They went with us to chemotherapy and kept us company during the many hours we spent at the treatment center. They gave us their favorite books to read, helped us pick out our wigs, supplied warm hats for our bald heads, and kept in touch throughout the long months of our treatment. Sympathetic neighbors offered sleeping rooms to the out-of-town family and friends who traveled to Larry's funeral.

Much of this generosity was unexpected. There may have been people who disappointed us when we had cancer, but more than a few surprised us with their kindness. People we barely knew and people we hadn't seen in ages came out of the woodwork to wish us well. Current and former students rose to the occasion, too. As Leon said at one of our meetings, "the discovery of what people, some of whom are relative strangers, are capable of and how they express it was very uplifting, really, just very uplifting." It was humbling to learn that so many individuals cared about what was happening to us.

We aren't all that religious ourselves, but were moved by the many people who said they were praying for us. Patty considers herself a lapsed Catholic, yet she remains a spiritual person, "holding her arms open to the graces and prayers that people offer." When she had cancer, she was more than willing to wear the five Catholic saint medals one of her sisters gave her for protection. And we were honored when people donated money in our names or dedicated their cancer fundraising efforts to us. Patty's and Larry's families went all out in this regard. They organized a team for a breast cancer walk and raised $8,000 in contributions. Some of the money came from donations collected in a Wal-Mart parking lot, where Patty's daughter and her daughter's partner set up a table. On the table they put a poster showing Patty, smiling and bald from chemotherapy, and a sign saying, "This is my Mom! She has breast cancer! You must donate!" When she found out about this, Patty was slightly embarrassed—she hoped no one had posted the scene on Facebook! Yet, she was also deeply touched by their generosity, and knew they had acted out of love.

Former cancer patients were also immensely helpful. Most of the people who claimed to know what we were going through did not, but former patients were genuine cancer experts. They knew a lot about the medical side of the disease and passed on information no one else had given us. More importantly, they knew about the personal side of cancer. They had been through a similar crisis and could tell us how they coped. As Art reports in his chapter on support groups, not all former patients are in touch with their previous fears and desires. For some, it is too threatening to go back to that awful time. But we were lucky enough to speak with several former patients, as well as former caregivers, who knew just what we needed. Attuned to our situations, these mentors offered priceless wisdom during our own cancer struggles.

TOWARD SEEING AND HEARING

We wish we could say we have become experts in responding to cancer, but we haven't. We still have a hard time finding the right words to say to people facing cancer. Yet, we did learn some valuable things. A great deal of harm could be avoided if everyone kept a few points in mind when interacting with cancer patients and caregivers.

First, do not withdraw when cancer hits someone you know. It is far better to reach out than to remain silent. Simple messages like,

"I'm thinking of you" are often enough. On the other hand, "caring silently from a distance"⁵ is, frankly, useless.

Second, when you do get in touch, put some thought into your words and actions. Good intentions are not enough. Simplistic and unsubstantiated advice does more harm than good. Stories of miracle cures aren't especially helpful, nor are claims that you know what someone is going through. Pay attention to the people dealing with illness, and let them guide the conversation. Don't try to take control or interrupt when they are talking. Just be there and listen to what's on their minds. And check in from time to time, for the long weeks during and after treatment get very lonely.

Third, remember that this is another person's catastrophe, not yours. It isn't fair to expect patients and caregivers to console you. The situation calls for empathy, not a discussion of your own problems and fears. Cancer is physically and emotionally overwhelming, and people dealing with cancer have more than enough to handle without worrying about you. Find someone else you can talk to about your feelings, don't impose them on people in the midst of a cancer ordeal.

Cancer is an occasion for real human contact, an opportunity for moral engagement in ordinary life. It is impossible to exaggerate the amount of sustenance we drew from people who reached out to us when we faced cancer. We still feel great warmth and affection for them. They are our role models as we try to help others forced to deal with this disease.

Too many people miss the opportunity to be part of meaningful cancer interactions. The missed opportunities are losses for everyone. We've said a lot about the losses to patients and caregivers, but there are losses to others, too. People untouched by life's troubles lose an opportunity to visit territory they will occupy someday. Better to start seeing and hearing its residents now, than to be thrust in later, completely unprepared.

Notes

1. Anton Chekhov, "Gooseberries," in *The Essential Tales of Chekhov*, ed. Richard Ford (Hopewell, New Jersey: Ecco Press, 1998), 266–74, 270.

2. Chemo Chicks, "Excuse Me?" Retrieved January 30, 2011, from http://www. chemochicks.com/excuse_me.htm. Journalist Christopher Hitchens, recently diagnosed with advanced cancer, describes a few of his "excuse me" moments in "Miss Manners and the Big C," *Vanity Fair* (Dec. 2010). Retrieved January

30, 2010, from http://www.vanityfair.com/culture/features/2010/12/hitchens-201012

3. Arthur W. Frank, *At the Will of the Body: Reflections on Illness* (Boston: Houghton Mifflin, 1991, 2nd ed., 2002), 64.

4. Elisa Albert, *Dahlia* (New York: Free Press, 2008), 70.

5. Frank, *At the Will of the Body*, 104.

Support, Advocacy, and the Selves of People with Cancer

Arthur W. Frank

I fell in love with support groups in the fall of 1992, five years after my treatment for cancer. I was in the exercise room of an airport hotel in Houston. The heat outside, along with the bleakness of the landscape—perfectly square blocks, every inch paved, dotted with warehouses and hotels—made the indoor treadmill seem like a good idea. It was a fairly small room, and I got to talking to a woman on the treadmill next to me. Like me, she was in the hotel for a conference sponsored by the M. D. Anderson Cancer Center's patient support organization. I was going to give the closing keynote speech of the conference; it was the first big hotel ballroom speaking event in the phase of my career that followed publication of my memoir, *At the Will of the Body*.[1]

After my fellow exerciser and I established we were both there for the conference—which had pretty much taken over the hotel—she said something that completely changed my perception of cancer survivorship, group affiliation, and myself. She said, with a vaguely apologetic tone, "I didn't actually have cancer myself; I'm here as a support person." The key word for me was *actually*, although this happened almost twenty years ago, and she might have used a different word to qualify her status as not having had cancer herself. What mattered is how, in that hotel for the duration of that conference, a normal assumption about identity was reversed.

At that moment, I realized what it had meant to spend the previous five years telling people I had had cancer. I had always been the one offering my history of cancer as something odd about myself. But, in the strangely configured demographics of that hotel for those three days, the foreground and background had switched. Those who had *not* had cancer were accountable for what became, in that very particular time and place, the oddity of their histories.

Hearing that woman express her need to qualify her identity, I felt the enormous relief of being what linguists call the unmarked category; that is, the identity assumed to be normal, which need not account for itself, as opposed to all the marked categories that constitute some version of difference from the unmarked. *She* had to explain her presence; I belonged there. And belonging felt good. It had been a long time.

One of the several ways in which our cancer ethics group is distinctly unrepresentative is that I seem to have been the only member to participate in support groups. My own participation involved a mixture of professional interest and personal need—the story I have just told suggests the layers of my participation. This chapter uses my own erratic and multilayered involvements as an opening to ask what is necessary about support groups but also how they can be either limiting or actually damaging. I begin by asking how the particular form of association known as "support groups" comes to be.

ORGANIZING TIME AND SPACE

Clinics and support groups are similar in at least this respect: each is an organization of time and space, in which a particular identity—a sense of self—is both made possible and required. The great Russian philosopher and literary critic Mikhail Bakhtin (1895–1975) described what he called the *chronotope*, based on his understanding of Einstein's theory of relativity. Bakhtin understood chronotopes as "the intrinsic connectedness of temporal and spatial relationships ... the inseparability of space and time."[2]

Both clinics and support groups take place in physical spaces, and both organize those spaces according to principles of duration—how long the activities understood to take place in those spaces will last. Clinical space is inseparable from duration: the time strictly allotted for appointments and procedures, and the expandable time of waiting. Support groups are also organized around the duration of meetings, or at the conference in Houston, the length of sessions, speeches, meals, and breaks. All of this is fairly obvious, but then Bakhtin says something more interesting, if opaque. "The image of man is always intrinsically chronotopic," he writes.[3]

I understand Bakhtin to mean that how we humans are able to understand ourselves—our sense of identity or self—depends crucially on the temporal and spatial organizations in which we live. The chronotope does not simply enable people to organize their activity; more important, it generates the consciousness of those who engage in that activity. Our image of ourselves is chronotopic because we have our being within and according to specific organizations of time and space, and both clinics and support groups are potent forms of such organizations.

Support groups take place in defined spaces, or more accurately, spaces that are generally redefined for use by the group: small conference rooms, church basements, hotel ballrooms. The activity, "support," has a duration, generally specified in advance. What this chronotope accomplishes is the gestalt switch I reflectively appreciated in that hotel exercise room, when my companion designated *not* having had cancer as the marked identity. Support groups organize time and space around a principle of the unmarked identity being the cancer survivor, that identity ranging from newly diagnosed to living in stable remission for decades. People who have not had cancer attend meetings to support the ill person or contribute specialized expertise to the group, but their identity is the marked category. Their presence must be accounted for, while ours is natural and entitled.

The ethical import is no less considerable for being subtle. I understand *ethics* in a broadly Aristotelian sense of seeking to live a good life, seeking what Aristotle calls human *flourishing*. Let me cite not Aristotle but Leon Kass, writing to introduce the collection of readings that the President's Council on Bioethics assembled during Kass's tenure as chair. He locates ethics in "the need to uphold human dignity and the many ways of doing and feeling and being in the world that make human life rich, deep, and fulfilling."[4] Kass proceeds to write that the Council understood bioethics not as based on biology, but as "an ethics in the service of *bios*—of a life lived humanly, a course of life lived not merely physiologically, but also mentally, culturally, politically, and spiritually."[5] My argument is that we humans live our mental, cultural, political, and spiritual lives within chronotopes, particularly organizations of time and space. Our possibility of being *ethical*, in Kass's generous sense, depends on being in a chronotope, because the chronotope *enables certain forms of action* and discourages other forms of action.

Both clinics and support groups, as chronotopes, enable living with illness as an expected, recognized, unmarked category—but there the similarity stops. In the clinic, the patient is subjected to a temporal and spatial ordering that is imposed upon him or her. As any number of social scientific studies and first-person illness narratives attest, the clinic reduces the patient to a disease that is the object of technical attention and intervention. In Kass's terms, life is merely physiological. The ideal of support groups is to reverse that process: to mark spaces and temporal durations in which people can pursue what Kass calls "a life lived humanly . . . not merely physiologically." But support groups are human institutions, and the reality often falls short of the ideal.

QUALIFYING SUPPORT

I came to be suspicious of support groups one evening when a local group invited me give a talk; this was also during the first years after *At the Will of the Body*. Before my talk, there were various group announcements: future meetings and social events, as well as personal news about members. A long-standing member of the group was reported to be in the hospital, her remission from cancer having ended. The announcement was punctuated with sighs and sidelong glances, conveying the unspoken message that this woman was most probably dying. The chairperson said that she welcomed visitors and then editorialized on that welcome, adding that the dying woman was "still the same old [person's name], laughing and joking." The necessity of that addendum seemed obvious: Even in a support group, the potential contagion of dying had to be neutralized. Maybe this woman felt like laughing and joking; I couldn't know. But the point was that the group had to be reassured. Visiting had to be made safe. Support clearly had its limits. The chronotope of the support group reorganized aspects of the image of cancer, but not so much of the fear.

Months later, another experience gave me a phrase that perfectly articulated my reservations about the group. It literally was a dark and stormy night—miserable early-winter weather—when the group was scheduled to meet. I called another group member who had mobility problems and asked if she would like a ride that night. She thanked me but said she had decided to pass on the meeting. "I can't take the *enforced hilarity*," she said to me, by way of explanation. I knew she was right. From that moment, I probably attended the group more from professional interest than with any expectation of personal support.

SUPPORT WRIT LARGE

The most physically expansive chronotopes of support—organizing the most space for the longest duration and endowing those within that time/space with a particular image—are civic run/walk/bike events that raise funds for what is often glossed as "the cure," a phrase endowing the chronotope with a distinctive goal. And the self-evident value of this goal, in turn, validates the chronotope.

One year on the national day of the multi-city run dedicated to breast cancer, I was in Montreal speaking to a hospital-based support and advocacy group. A member of the group gave me a ride to the run; as I recall, she had been diagnosed and treated fairly recently. In those events, runners wear bibs that not only have their race numbers, but also provide space to write the names of people with cancer whom the runner wishes to support or remember. So, before this race, I was writing on my bib the names of the women closest to me who had breast cancer. Some were living and some had died.

As I kept on adding names, my friend stopped whatever she was doing and watched me. "So many names," she said, as if she were realizing something for the first time. And over the years, I thought, you too will add more names. If that young woman remained active in the support group, the names she wrote on her race bib would come more quickly. But even if she left the world of support groups, there would be names enough.

Then to assemble with all the other people wearing their bibs, and to spend the duration of the race passing by many names and being passed by many others, that is an act of public witness to what is too often kept from view.

My home city of Calgary is built around a river, and the course for the last such event I participated in went up one side of the river and back the other side. As these events include participants of all fitness levels, it was possible to look across the river and see, spread out, the thousands of people who were there. The great sociologist Emile Durkheim observed how rituals effect a merging of selves into a collective, so that the sense of individual separation is subsumed.[6] On that spring day, as the sun shone on the river and all those people memorialized lives lived with breast cancer, it was possible to feel part of something that was truly grand—a wholeness that holds each part.

But I did not stay for the speeches after the race, because I did not want to be made painfully aware of what, I knew from experience, would not be spoken. In the crowd after the race I saw a friend whom

I had known long before either of us had cancer. She was now in a wheelchair, the progression of her disease having made walking difficult. She had been deeply involved in the survivorship community, but at least in previous years, the ceremonies would make no acknowledgment of lives like hers. There might be cheers for people in treatment who were running surrounded by their support teams, but the whole event was about sustaining a version of hope that excluded the realities of decline in wheelchairs and all-too-imminent death.

The post-race ceremonies would be dominated by announcements of how much money had been raised and brief techno-science talks by cancer researchers whose work was funded by such events. Nikolas Rose and Carlos Novas, scholars who specialize in bodies, health and regulation, and systems of thought, coin the usefully descriptive phrase, "the political economy of hope," which is a perfect description of such events. "Hope," they write, "thus ties together personal biographies, the aspirations that patients share for better treatments or a cure, and the campaigns of patients' groups to achieve particular goals."[7] The triumphalism of the post-race talks seeks to reassure the audience that biological life, despite risks of cancer, "is no longer blind destiny, or even foreseen but implacable fate," as Rose and Novas write.[8] The political economy of hope is that through *participation*—comprising running, donating, and consuming—life becomes less risky and more "knowable, mutable, improvable, eminently manipulable." Post-race talks were all testimonials to how cancer risk was being rendered knowable; how techno-medicine was manipulating biology in the cause of improving lives. The other crucial element in the political economy of hope is that *hope* is inscribed under a corporate logo, and therein lies its political economy. "But of course," Rose and Novas observe, "this activity is to take a specific, brand-related form."[9] The spirit of a "Run for the Cure" was never expressed more succinctly.[10]

Participation offers control of biological destiny, but participation also induces and indeed requires acceptance of the "brand-related form" that organizes the chronotope of the event: its time and space, sense of purpose, and parameters of acceptable expression. In sum, participants have to become what the event requires them to be: hopeful according to a particular version of corporatized techno-science. And then there is what the event excludes.

"Of course," Rose and Novas continue, "the other side of hope is undoubtedly anxiety, fear, and even dread at what one's biological future, or that of those one cares for, might hold."[11] In the post-race ebullience about how medical science was conquering cancer, I would hear only the erasure of the names of the dead that were on our bibs. Cancer would be formulated in the genre of *romance*: a story of humanity's collective over-coming of adversity. Maybe my skeptical response to telling cancer stories within this genre is only my problem. *Why*, I ask myself at such moments, do I always need a counterbalance of tragedy? To which one reasonable answer is: to honor the dead and to respect the holes in the lives of those left behind by those deaths. During the run itself, I could feel those narratives of romance and tragedy were in brief, fragile balance. But afterward, hope shows its foundation in political economy.

ALLOWING DEATH

There can be memorials within festivals. In 1996, I attended a meeting of the National Coalition for Cancer Survivorship (NCCS) in Albuquerque, New Mexico. The group was just about to move its national headquarters to Washington, D.C. in order to be better positioned to engage in political advocacy work. At the closing dinner, before speeches that included one by the National Cancer Institute's medical director, the evening began with a reading of the names of members who had died during the previous year. After each name, a bell was rung. Then someone who had known that person spoke briefly about him or her. It was an extraordinary ritual of personal and collective remembrance. It also brought everyone back to the basic reality that whatever the NCCS did, people would *die* of cancer.

The NCCS memorial seemed so right to me—so *necessary*—because my own treatment for cancer proceeded in parallel with the treatment of two people who were especially close to me: the wife of a colleague who was diagnosed when I was, and my mother-in-law, who had been in and out of remission for years. They both died about eighteen months after my treatment ended. It has always seemed to me to be nothing more than blind fate that I should have been the one to have lived; call it the luck of histology. My own survival has always been, for me, anything but a triumph. Instead, it is an ongoing memorial.

At the NCCS meeting, when death was spoken, its anxiety diminished. The living could accept the luck of their own survival.

FROM SUPPORT TO ADVOCACY

The NCCS is one of many groups that offer peer support but also engage in forms of public advocacy. In some hospital-based groups, advocacy is limited to raising money for projects ranging from building patient and family lounges to funding research and clinical positions. The NCCS engages in political advocacy; at the time of that meeting in Albuquerque, one of its singular achievements was successfully lobbying government officials to include cancer as one of the conditions covered by the Americans with Disabilities Act, which provided protection against job loss as a result of illness.

Groups have different positions along a continuum of advocacy, from what could be called constructive support to adversarial activism. The former raise funds for local projects; the latter lobby for increased government funding for cancer programs or reallocation of funds to such programs. Both, however, accept without question the premises of biomedicine and its assertion of an achievable cure.

A different form of adversarial activism merges politics inspired by feminism, AIDS activism, and radical ecology movements. Such groups criticize how mainstream cancer advocacy evades and obscures the role its corporate sponsors may be playing in causing cancer as a by-product of their products and the environmental degradation caused by their production practices. The sociologist Maren Klawiter's ethnographic study of cancer activism in the San Francisco area examines the politics and shifting structures of these groups in detail. In one chapter, Klawiter describes changes in support group resources through the history of a woman she calls Clara Larson, who was diagnosed with breast cancer first in 1979 and again in 1997. Klawiter interviewed her in 1998, while she was recovering from a stem-cell transplant. "The difference," Klawiter writes, "is that in 1979 Clara looked for political community but was unable to find it. In 1997, she felt called upon to justify her lack of political involvement."[12] Differences in what form of support is available predispose differences in what identities people can take up. But there is the finest of lines between making an identity available and prescribing that identity.

PRESCRIBING SELVES

Klawiter quotes Clara Larson's declaration: "Nobody understands this experience unless they've gone through it."[13] That is the single most cited reason for support groups to exist. But Larson's statement, by itself, suggests a homogeneity of perspective that does not exist. The tension in support groups is between members' different understandings of what they have been through and what helped them get through it.

Time intensifies this tension; group members just starting to go through treatment, or even still in diagnosis, have different needs than do those who look back on having gone through cancer years, or even decades, earlier.

The group I once attended has now ceased to exist. The multiple causes of its demise, so far as I can tell, included a combination of leadership, demographics, and the Internet. Groups require a stable core of people who book the room, bring the refreshments, set up the chairs at the start and fold them at the end, schedule speakers, and, in many cancer support groups, pair peer volunteers with newly diagnosed patients who call the group asking for help. An inescapable problem of group maintenance is that these core volunteers get older and remain committed to keeping the group organized as it always has been. Younger members find that organization fails to provide a venue for the kind of service they hope to offer (although that service is often not well defined in their imaginations). When the Internet came along, support went virtual and dissatisfied members went online to find what they were looking for. But I quit attending my own group before the group quit meeting, and here is my last story, telling why.

The group began each meeting according to a template that the Founder, whose charismatic force persisted years after her death, had learned in her training elsewhere and imported. Much like a recovery group, each participant would introduce himself or herself, saying at least his or her name, date and nature of diagnosis, and present treatment status (if any). The introduction ended with a ritual statement of "I'm fine."

Everyone at the meeting was supposed to be fine; not without problems, but fine. Except, one night, a recently diagnosed woman came to the group, and no one told her that she was supposed to be fine. So, after she told us her diagnosis, she began to cry, which is what people often do when they have recently learned they have cancer. Neither group member sitting next to her moved to comfort her. Instead, the woman who was next in the order of introductions—one of the core organizers and someone long in remission—abruptly began introducing herself. She did this with particular brevity and assertion, ending with an especially forceful statement of "And I'm fine!" At least as I heard it, the tears were drowned out. And I knew it was my last meeting as anything like a member, even though the sociological part of me had considerable sympathy for the long-standing member. She was doing what she felt she had to, to sustain the group as she knew it.

People hold their own during cancer, as in life generally, by becoming deeply invested in the configuration of attitudes, expressive possibilities, and practical actions that constitute how they have held their lives together during crisis—or how a support group has led these people to recollect how they held their lives together, memory being subject to constant reinvention. Personal investment then often entails projecting their way of living onto others, in whom they see an image of their former selves, when their lives were upended by cancer. A great deal that is called *support* consists of that projection, much of which may be quite useful to the other person, but some of which grates. The long-standing member who cut in on the new member was not simply enforcing terms of membership; she was defending a narrative she lives by—a version of self that she truly believes others will sooner or later be better off adopting. I am no less invested in the stories that make up my way of living with cancer. But, as I form myself and relate to those around me, I might have available more stories than this woman has, which is not a trivial difference in what we each project onto others.[14]

Sociologists have produced multiple studies of how support groups structure the experiential narrative that members are allowed to tell and, very quickly, come to regard as their own, which they are—therein lies the duality of anyone's sense of self. Leslie Irvine studied a self-help group called Codependents Anonymous. She observes that, although groups do enforce varying degrees of narrative conformity, "stories of the self" are not "capriciously cobbled together."[15] Stories told in groups have traction insofar as they blend seamlessly into stories that become people's "internal conversations." Irvine's conclusion is a good summary of the sociological view of the self that I find inescapably compelling: "We cannot 'do' selfhood alone, but it must work when we are alone if it is to work in front of others."[16] In other words, we humans always learn the stories we regard as "our own" within the institutionally organized chronotopes in which we spend our lives.

To be clear, the issue here is not some kind of false consciousness. Institutions and groups do not colonize a self that would be authentic if it were left to itself. There is no self except in contact with others. The idea of the self that is most relevant to support groups is Charles Taylor's *dialogical authenticity*. "No one acquires the languages needed for self-definition on their own," Taylor writes.[17] Support groups are one scene—or one chronotope, to use Bakhtin's more precise term—in which people learn a language that they hope will be sufficiently rich to express what cancer requires expressing: all the anger, suffering, regret, mourning, love, and more than occasional joy to which people's accounts of illness testify. If the expressive languages that most support groups teach their members can be found lacking, that criticism applies equally to families, schools, religious organizations, and all the other institutions in which people learn to tell stories of the self. That lack is also known as the human condition.

LANGUAGE, SUPPORT, AND THE GOOD LIFE

The case for support groups comes to this: The language of medicine will always be too thin as an *expressive* language. Medical language is designed to describe pathology as precisely as possible. While we might well ask health care workers to have a richer expressive language in their relationships with patients, those workers will—with enormous individual variation—remain limited by what makes them useful as professionals.[18] Patients need to talk to people who live illness outside the clinic, responding to all the relational contingencies that enrich life as a whole. As long as there is cancer, there will need to be support groups.

The problem of support groups—their tendency to impose identities and circumscribe agendas for action—is complementary to their necessity: People join because they lack resources to reconstitute identities as cancer survivors, and they lack agendas for action. As long as there are groups, those who organize the meetings, including booking the room, making the coffee, and unfolding and restacking the chairs, will project the particular expressive possibilities in which they are deeply invested, leaving potential members to sort out whether that language is appropriate to their lives, with its tastes, recognitions (political as well as personal), and affiliations. This problem seems to be no less an issue for virtual support groups, which are marked by constant schisms over the appropriateness of how the group is being moderated—but those stories go beyond my experience, which sets the parameters of this chapter.

All of these stories of support groups are true, insofar as I try to tell each story according to my memory of what I experienced. My intention is not for one to trump any other. The issue is neither synthesis nor judgment; rather, it is living with how any chronotope has a multiplicity of effects on those who inhabit it for long enough. Appreciating multiplicity does not mean refusing to take sides; it does mean trying to see as clearly as possible what is at stake on the other side.

Here, we return to what I remarked earlier in this chapter about ethics as more than biological existence. In a post-Enlightenment, multicultural world, we necessarily live with competing versions of the *good life*; no one version has absolute priority. I understand the Aristotelian ideal of *flourishing* to be a matter of holding open the issue of which version of the good life I am called to live. And especially, with what variation I am called to live differently from the template versions of a good life in which numerous entities—voluntary, corporate, and often blended voluntary-corporatized—seek to enroll me.

Support groups are, on my understanding of ethics, deeply ethical, because their issues involve the terms on which people will relate to each other in the quest for a good life. Yet, attempts to imagine an ethics of support groups must keep in mind both the sociological realities of group formation and maintenance, as well the existential drama of the human condition. At the end of the day, we can hope only that most people find enough of what they need, and that those who do not will go on to form new groups.

Notes

1. Arthur W. Frank, *At the Will of the Body: Reflections on Illness* (Boston: Houghton Mifflin, 1991; reprint edition with a new Afterword, Mariner Books, 2002).
2. Mikhail Bakhtin, "Form of Time and Chronotope in the Novel: Notes Toward a Historical Poetics," in M. M. Bakhtin, *The Dialogic Imagination: Four Essays*. Translated by Caryl Emerson and Michael Holquist (Austin: University of Texas Press, 1981), 84. Brackets in original.
3. Bakhtin, "Form of Time," 85.
4. Leon Kass, "Being Human: An Introduction," in *Being Human: Core Readings in the Humanities* (New York: Norton, 2004), xx.
5. Kass, "Being Human," xx–xxi.
6. Emile Durkheim, *The Elementary Forms of Religious Life*. Translated by Joseph Ward Swain (New York: Free Press, 1965 [1912]).
7. Nikolas Rose and Carlos Novas, "Biological Citizenship," in *Global Assemblages: Technology, Politics, and Ethics as Anthropological Problems*, ed. Aihwa Ong and Stephen Collier (Oxford: Blackwell, 2005), 452.
8. Rose and Novas, "Biological Citizenship," 442.
9. Rose and Novas, "Biological Citizenship," 447. The quotation refers specifically to Prozac, but the argument is intended to be generalized, as I do here; cf. n. 7.
10. "Race for the Cure" is the trademarked brand of the Susan G. Komen Foundation. For extensive discussion of these events as a nexus of corporate, civic, and medical interests, see Samantha King, *Pink Ribbons, Inc.*

(Minneapolis: University of Minnesota Press, 2006). King fills in the details of Rose and Novas's observation that the political economy of hope depends on how "the hope for the innovation that will treat or cure stimulates the circuits of investment" (n. 7, p. 442). My own participation was in Canadian "Run for the Cure" events, that slight difference between names expressing some national difference. Other differences between the "Race" and the "Run" events seem to be of scale only.

11. Rose and Novas, "Biological Citizenship," 442.
12. Maren Klawiter, *The Biopolitics of Breast Cancer: Changing Cultures of Disease and Activism* (Minneapolis: University of Minnesota Press, 2008), 243.
13. Klawiter, *The Biopolitics of Breast Cancer*, 235.
14. For an extended argument on the importance of having more stories available, see Arthur W. Frank, *Letting Stories Breathe: A Socio-Narratology* (Chicago: University of Chicago Press, 2010), Chapter 5.
15. Leslie Irvine, *Codependent Forevermore: The Invention of Self in a Twelve Step Group* (Chicago: University of Chicago Press, 1999), 63. See also Frank, *Letting Stories Breathe*, "Institutional Emplotment of Individuals' Stories," 134–38.
16. Irvine, *Codependent Forevermore*, 63.
17. Charles Taylor, *The Malaise of Modernity* (Concord, Ontario: House of Anansi Press, 1991), 33. [Printed in the United States as *The Ethics of Authenticity*, Harvard University Press.]
18. A classic expression of this critique of medical language is Elliot Mishler, *The Discourse of Medicine: Dialectics of Medical Interviews* (Norwood N.J.: Ablex Publishing Corporation, 1984). See also Arthur W. Frank, *The Wounded Storyteller: Body, Illness, and Ethics* (Chicago: University of Chicago Press, 1995). For what expressive possibilities are available within medical language, see Arthur W. Frank, *The Renewal of Generosity: Illness, Medicine, and How to Live* (Chicago; University of Chicago Press, 2004).

CHAPTER 13

Cancer and Mortality

Making Time Count

Leon R. Kass

Strength and dignity are her clothing, and she laughs at the time to come. [1]
So teach us to number our days that we may get a heart of wisdom. [2]

All human beings are mortal, and nearly all of us know it. But, for most of us, through much of our lives, this knowledge remains largely below the level of consciousness. The arrival of cancer—in our own life or the life of our loved ones—shatters this congenial forgetfulness. Sleeping knowledge of personal finitude is rudely awakened, generally with massive consequences for everyday life. More than any other illness, cancer is a brutal reminder not only that we are *really* going to die, but also that we—or someone we love—will be, from this day forward, "*more* mortal" than others. This chapter, written as my wife of fifty years undergoes chemotherapy for the fourth time in her (our) sixth year of living with ovarian cancer, offers some reflections on how this awareness affects the way we do, can, and (perhaps) should live. It also touches on questions—humanly less important but professionally pertinent—about the field of bioethics and how it should be practiced.

The approach of bioethics to cancer must be, at bottom, concerned with the intersection of ethics and mortality. When cancer appears, the largest ethical question, "How to live?" comes under intense pressure from the now-impossible-to-ignore threat of inevitable death. What happens as a result of this confrontation is no trivial matter, neither for life as lived nor for life as the subject of ethical reflection. For if nothing concentrates the guilty mind like an impending hanging, nothing concentrates the ordinary mind like a diagnosis of cancer: It reminds us daily of the disproportion between the boundless aspirations and timeless longings of the human soul and the finitude and frailty of our living body. This "discovery" should, of course, not be news to anyone seriously interested in ethics, inasmuch as the moral life depends altogether on this disjunction. Were we not embodied and hence mortal creatures, harboring both unlimited desires and fears of death, there would be little need for—or possibility of—self-restraint, self-command, and ethical instruction regarding rightful and noble conduct.

Ordinary bioethics, as professionally practiced today, largely steers clear of these deep issues of living with, and against, mortality. Like medicine, whose moral dilemmas it seeks to address, bioethics is largely a reactive discipline. It takes its bearings not from life as ordinarily lived at home, work, and play, but from life as reconceived through encounters with the institutions of science, technology, and medicine.

Responding to problems generated by technological progress in biomedical settings, and focused on issues of autonomy, distributive justice, and risks of bodily harm, professional bioethics today pays little attention to the profound existential issues implicit in the human life cycle, including the inevitability of decline, suffering, finitude, and loss—matters which are not bioethical problems to be solved, but rather human challenges to be faced and borne. For this reason, bioethics to date has had very little to contribute to the deepest concerns of persons afflicted with cancer and their families, concerns that are neither medical nor narrowly bioethical but rather existential and spiritual. Still, I dare to hope that thoughtful attention to the life world of persons with cancer and their families may yet contribute to a deepening of bioethical reflection and practice. At the center of such reflection must be the question of mortality—what it means, and how to face it.

THE VIRTUES OF MORTALITY

Nearly thirty years ago, having already spent some fifteen years on concrete practical bioethical issues of death and dying (including defining death, terminating treatment, and allowing to die), I tried my hand at a general meditation on the relation between mortality and morality.

Although admitting that I might not know what I was talking about and that, in any case, time would teach me my lessons (it has!), I boldly wrote about the blessings of mortality—or at least, the blessings of *awareness* of one's *own* mortality—for *how* we live. Among the benefits I cited: prospects for increased engagement and seriousness, greater appreciation of things beautiful and beloved, increased incentives to spend one's life on things that matter, and willingness to invest generously in children and grandchildren, rather than selfishly only in oneself.

In that earlier meditation, I also argued for the deep connection between mortality and moral excellence or virtue:

> To be mortal means that it is possible to give one's life, not only in one moment, say on the field of battle, but also in the many other ways in which we are able in action to rise above attachment to survival. Through moral courage, endurance, greatness of soul, generosity, devotion to justice—in acts great and small—we rise above our mere creatureliness, spending the precious coinage of the time of our lives for the sake of the noble and the good and the holy. . . . [Y]et for this nobility, vulnerability and mortality are the necessary conditions. The immortals cannot be noble.[3]

In support of these conclusions, I invoked evidence from Homer—shown me by my wife—quoting Odysseus' speech to the nymph Calypso, in which he turns down her offer to be lord of her household and immortal:

> Goddess and queen, do not be angry with me. I myself know that all you say is true and that circumspect Penelope can never match the impression you make for beauty and stature. She is mortal after all, and you are immortal and ageless. But even so, what I want and all my days I pine for is to go back to my house and see that day of my homecoming. And if some god batters me far out on the wine-blue water, I will endure it, keeping a stubborn spirit inside me, for already I have suffered much and done much hard work on the waves and in the fighting.[4]

Interpreting in my own name, I commented, "To suffer, to endure, to trouble oneself for the sake of home, family, community, and genuine friendship, is truly to live, and is the clear choice of this exemplary mortal. . . . Immortality is a kind of oblivion, like death itself."

I can no longer read this speech of Odysseus with dry eyes. Indeed, my recent experience as the spouse of someone struggling with a serious cancer has forced me to reconsider my thinking about this subject. With respect only to myself, I am still inclined to affirm the benefits of finitude for thinking of my own future. But I am astonished to discover my earlier stupidity in adopting a purely self-centered view of the question and in failing to think at all about the mortality of the one I love.

Although, as I will later indicate, there are indeed certain "benefits" from recognizing acutely that we two no longer have world enough and time, I repent of my earlier praise of mortality when it comes to her: there is nothing good to be said in favor of the finitude of my beloved. Her innocent suffering (psychic as well as somatic) strikes me as cosmic injustice; the idea of her possible extinction fills me with horror; and, more selfishly, the hard-to-banish thought that I am going to lose her drowns me periodically in waves of anticipatory grief, with not a glimmer of redemptive good anticipated. The greater the love, the worse the prospect—and, assuredly, worse yet the fact—of my beloved's annihilation.

"CHOOSING" CANCER?

None of the above insights, it is true, are specifically tied to cancer. Other diseases can surely teach these lessons. Why, even a brief reflection on the wrinkles of age—if they are not Botoxed away—makes for melancholy awareness that one of us will lose immensely by living left behind. As we approached our recently attained three score and ten, both my wife and I were increasingly aware that we were living on borrowed time and that they were shooting at us. We persist in hoping and praying that the lender will be merciful and that we may continue to dodge "their" bullets. But a recurrent bout or a steadily progressive course of cancer changes the outlook, rubbing our noses in the fact that time is now really all too short, and that, in the script of our life together, suffering, separation, and sorrow will get the last words.

Yet, when the demands of care and the voices of anxiety abate for a time, the reflective mind, stepping back, can discover that even these grim facts are open to competing evaluations, especially when one considers the alternative possibilities that Act V might have in store for us. When the President's Council on Bioethics was examining the ethics of caregiving in our aging society, with special attention to persons with dementia and other impairments that make it impossible for them to care for themselves,[5] Dr. Joanne Lynn made a presentation at a staff meeting that I will never forget. She began as follows: "How many of you would like to die of cancer?" In our group of ten, most of whom were under thirty-five years old, only one hand went up. She next asked, "Okay, so how many of you would like to die of major organ failure, say, of chronic congestive heart failure or chronic obstructive pulmonary disease (emphysema)?" No hands were raised. The same negative response followed her third invitation: "And how many of you would like to die after a prolonged period of debility, enfeeblement, and dementia, lasting perhaps up to a decade?"

With nine choices still to be voiced, Dr. Lynn asked again: "Okay, *now* how many of you would like to die of cancer?" People having caught on, there were a few more takers this time around—especially after Dr. Lynn pointed out that most Americans today die in one of these three major ways: roughly 20% from cancer, 20% from major organ failure, and a whopping 40% following an extended period of diminishment, both in body and in mind. (The remaining 20% of us die from one or another of dozens of less prevalent causes or trajectories.)

The question, "Of what do you want to die?" is idle, not to say foolish. We do not get to choose how we will meet our end. Indeed, death is *the* refutation of our proud belief that we are in charge of our lives, the noble lie that enables us to live with blind hopes and to walk with some confidence in this life. But the point of the question is not, in fact, about choice, but rather about wish and hope, and it therefore offers an interesting path to self-knowledge. Moreover, reflecting on this subject can have ethical implications, less for how we actually die, more for how we choose to live in the meantime, even when confronting cancer or other life-threatening illnesses. The "foolish" question not only puts us in mind of the certainty of our finitude; it reminds us that there are better and worse ways to leave this world, and, more to the point, it invites us to think about *why* we might prefer one form of dying to another, which is to say, one way of *living-while-dying* to another.

I confess that I was the person who raised his hand the first time Dr. Lynn offered us the "choice" to die of cancer—and I think I would have stuck to my preference even if the other options had included sudden death from heart attack or stroke. Having long meditated on this morbid subject, I had seen—or thought I had seen—the advantages of anticipating what is coming, of meeting an end that comes gradually without usually (as in Alzheimer's disease) losing one's powers of awareness, of having the opportunity to *make something* of the remaining time, of having time to heal human relations and to allow others to get used to our impending departure. Experience with cancer since that day has given me more than pause, as I will soon indicate, but these intuitions are not without some merit.

At the same time, I recognize that the preference I was expressing could not be widely shared, and not even when people see that there are, for most of us, only worse alternatives. That another person's fate is worse provides no remedy for my own. And only a fool would think cancer *for itself* something to be wished for.

People like me who want to have some advance warning of the final curtain, who desire a stretch of time to complete projects or put their affairs in order, want only the chronicity, not the malignancy, of cancer. No sensible person will embrace the cumulative and ever-increasing suffering involved, the ravaging of the body, or the inchoate feeling of being "possessed" by evil forces that are invisibly eating away at our powers and turning us into mere shells of our former selves. And notwithstanding the great progress that has been made in treating—and often "curing"—cancer over the past half-century (40% of Americans alive today will get the disease during their lifetime, but only half will succumb to it), few sensible people will cheerfully embrace the highly debilitating forms of treatment—not only surgery, but toxic chemotherapy and radiation—which are often harder to endure than the disease itself, and which a century hence, I am sure, will strike our descendants as barbaric. Yes, all human beings die, owing to some fatal disease or other, but dying of cancer really is different. The popular dread of cancer is anything but irrational.

It is true, and worth remembering, that cancer is not a single disease, and the term adheres to many different types of malignancy. These range from, say, glioblastoma multiforme, a insidiously growing and incurable brain tumor that can lead to death within weeks or even days of first diagnosis, to basal cell carcinoma, an easily detected cancer of the skin that is usually cured by simple surgical removal. In between are malignancies of varying degrees of invasiveness and aggression, responsiveness to treatments, and danger to life. Some of these cancers are now treated like other chronic illnesses, with patients going in and out of remission after being in and out of treatment, and many people known to have cancer live long enough to die of some other cause.

Variations in the natural history of the malignancy make for widely differing experiences, and "having cancer," therefore, will likely have a different meaning even for the same person, depending on *which* cancer he happens to get. (Rebecca Dresser and Norman Fost make this point in their earlier chapter, "Cancer Stereotypes.") Nevertheless, in most cases there appears to be something irreducibly common in being struck with this diagnosis, not in the biology of the disease but in the perception of its meaning. While we rely on doctors to deal with the cancer, we must ourselves struggle with its personal and human meaning, which we can glimpse with greater or lesser clarity or intensity as our experience with the disease goes through its various phases.

WHY CANCER IS MALIGNANT

As John Robertson describes in "Learning the Bad News," nothing can prepare you for the shock of the first diagnosis of the dread disease. My wife was in perfect health when her disease was first diagnosed: an abnormal mass found on annual gynecological examination, rendered more suspicious by sonographic and radiographic scans, and confirmed as malignant only at surgery. Although surgical and pathology reports agreed that the cancer had not yet spread (and thus, we were encouraged to believe, had been completely removed), chemotherapy was instituted for good measure, and we began to think in battle mode against mortality, caught between hope and fear.

That I tended more toward optimism and my wife more toward apprehension was not simply the product of our temperamental differences: It was, after all, *her* cancer and *her* life. She feared the hidden presence of deadly cells, the assassin's terror network that evaded the surgical strike. She also had to endure the ignominy of being a helpless victim, unable to fight back or to defend herself, reliant on doctors and nurses and harmful medicines to preserve her from the enemy within.

I too felt helpless and impotent, yet I had a different response. I gladly placed my trust in modern medicine and its practitioners. For my wife, however, the tools of modern medicine only made the outlook worse. The symptoms that the chemotherapy drugs produced—fatigue, nausea, hair loss, and the severe numbness and tingling in the feet and hands that doctors call neuropathy—were themselves anxiety-inducing and depressing harbingers of the very decline and decay that they were being used to prevent. The neuropathy was—and remains—especially troubling, as her every step is both physically uncomfortable and psychically disconcerting. Unfeeling and unsteady afoot, unable to walk without awareness of abnormality, she experiences a partial yet growing estrangement from terra firma.

The end of the initial regimen of chemotherapy brought its own new, and utterly unexpected, evils and fears. The potent pharmacological mercenaries had been dismissed, and it seemed that *no one* was then fighting for her life. Even more than before, she stood naked and alone before mortality: Death loomed larger when there appeared to be nothing barring the way. Reassurance from the doctor that gloomy thoughts and clinical depression are common, occurring generally within four to six weeks after the end of treatment, did not make them go away. The truth of our vulnerable situation could no longer be avoided: We were at the mercy of powers—and devils—invisible.

There were many reminders of cancer even after that first round of chemotherapy ended. Consciousness of her body would obtrude itself unpredictably yet often, sometimes with new aches or pains that raised anxieties about possible metastases, more often simply to destroy the comfortable lack of self-attention needed for any whole-hearted engagement in life's activities. Whatever the merits of self-consciousness in general, there can be no doubt that this sort of self-awareness is by itself terribly corrosive, even deadly, for life as it wants to be lived.

Beyond the direct hyperawareness of her body, made ill by the treatments, there was also the eerie feeling that her body was no longer fully hers. She was not only host to her mortal enemy. Worse, unlike potentially deadly bacteria who are invaders from outside, her cancer had sprung from her own body—from her organ of generation, no less— her own flesh had turned traitor, in league with annihilating evil. With cancer, the prospect of death is visualized not as an outside attacker with grim visage and scythe, but as incarnated in one's very being. Yes, everyone may know that we are born to death, that life is intrinsically, and not accidentally, mortal. But to *feel* the presence of death lurking within is, to say the least, extremely disconcerting. More than death by organ failure or progressive decay—"the parts just wore out from overuse"—or death from infection—"the invader was too powerful"— death from cancer feels more like a form of self-destruction.

If one is lucky, as my wife first was, remission supervenes, in her case lasting long enough to make us believe, foolishly, that the battle had been won. As the weeks and months passed, as each successive scan showed no recurrence of the disease, and the dark days of diagnosis and treatment began to recede into memory, we began to resume the kind of "thoughtless living" that we "enjoyed" before. We made plans with less uncertainty, we accepted obligations a year or two hence, we threw ourselves into our projects as before, maybe with even greater abandon. To be sure, the sense that we were blessed still to have one another, and in health, was never far from consciousness. But there was a return to "daily-ness" that comes naturally, with the risk of losing the edge that comes from having the grim reaper staring at you from your beloved's shoulders. To think too much of mortality is to fail to live, to think too little of it risks failing to live as fully and as richly as possible.

For my wife, truth to tell, intimations of mortality were never totally absent, not even in the heady late stages of the lengthy remission, when we dared to hope that she was cured. When asked, she would insist both that everything was different and that nothing was different. Although the activities and loves of her life remained the same, her outlook on life was different. If pressed, she would concede that the changes and new insights were not owed to the fact that the disease was cancer, rather than some other life-threatening illness. Nonetheless, the encounter with cancer and its treatment impressed her with the often-hidden truth about our life: that the time of our lives, unlike the time of the physicists, is a unidirectional arrow going forward. For us, there was no "going back" to some status quo ante, no matter how much our self-conception and dominant worldview denied this fact.

We tend to believe that we are in control, and if we do not like a path we have chosen, we can also get ourselves back to the origin, and choose a different one. During the period of remission, my wife seemed as free of ovarian cancer as she was the day I married her. Yet she—and also I—was not the same, not in body and not even in soul. Time and events write themselves into our existence; we rarely are aware of the fact. (I refer here not to a psychological fact, but an ontological one, yet one that the experience of potentially lethal illness may make conscious.)

In the end, my wife's cancer did not allow us to remain with such benign philosophical questions about living with mortality. Alas, after a three and a half year period of lying low, beneath detection, the cancer made a reappearance. Out of the blue. Recurrence with metastases, once again asymptomatic, discovered this time on periodic computed tomography (CT) scan. Now there is more and different chemotherapy to save her life by making her sick. There are new side effects, some bothersome, some dangerous. It is no longer possible to believe in a cure: The oncologist insensitively blurts it out explicitly ("Since we are not going for a cure"), by way of rationalizing his decision to postpone a scheduled treatment because her blood counts were not yet up to snuff.

The new medical mantra is "Ovarian cancer is a chronic disease," one for which we have many tools to knock it back into remission. Yet, we are also told, the periods of remission will be shorter and shorter. It becomes exceedingly difficult to keep persuading myself and my wife—who has ample reason not to be persuaded—that she is not under a sentence of death. Some people really are—and, equally important existentially, surely *feel* themselves to be—*more mortal* than others. The dark cloud that hangs over us now will never be seen to disappear.

LIVING WELL AND DYING WELL

The facts of suffering and likely separation through death are, for both of us, a curse. So, too, are the involuntarily recurring thoughts of what this loss will mean: for my wife, failure to see our lovely granddaughters grow into maturity, failure to give back to the world what she still has left to give, great regret at the thought of abandoning me to a lonely old age; for me, the overwhelming sadness of anticipated life without her at my side; for both of us, the poignant sense that we may be seeing this favorite place or doing this or that activity together for the last time.

And yet. And yet. The perception of death's growing nearness is—or at least *can* be and *has been*—in *some* respects also a blessing, because it makes the time we have together infinitely more precious. The joys of daily life together—indeed, the very *existence* of daily life *together*—are felt much more intensely: the sharing of meal preparations, daily walks in Rock Creek Park, re-reading aloud our favorite novels (all six of Jane Austen's), visiting with dear family and friends, finishing a book that we are writing together, watching old movies that we love, reminiscing about the days when the children were young or the adventures we have had, looking forward to our fiftieth anniversary and other family celebrations, telling each other—often—"Thank you for being here."

Despite the periodic bouts of sadness, we feel and gladly yield to the omnipresence of "the life force," which asserts itself in opposition to despair and which tries (for now, often successfully) to prevent the fear of the future from the destroying the wonderful possibilities of the present.[6] We take special inspiration from watching the coupled-off mallards and wood ducks greeting us daily on our wintry walks along Rock Creek, who refuse to be beaten by cold and frost, and who, swimming against the icy stream, instinctively celebrate the possibilities of life together in the midst of the world's inhospitality. We feel more strongly than ever before the miracle and majesty of love, which wells up from God knows where to suffuse every little touch, deed, and gesture.

Bad days have come and worse days may well be coming, but the ones we have been blessed to have—notwithstanding the ongoing trials and tribulations of chemotherapy—have allowed us to live and love in full, without remorse, without regret (except, I should confess, for the time stolen away from "life" to write this essay showing why every day should be lived in full). Thanks to these heightened powers of awareness and appreciation, we have been able to make something precious—in many ways, the best days of a very happy marriage—out of the curse that is cancer. No such "redemptive" possibility is available when death comes suddenly without warning, say from fatal heart attack or stroke, leaving life without its final act and the surviving spouse with only emptiness.

Sudden death or death following a prolonged period of enfeeblement and dementia also rule out the possibility of dying well, a matter once a topic of serious moral writing and attention. I mean here not only the sort of living well in the face of mortal illness, but facing bravely and beautifully the very last weeks and days of life. The deaths we most admire are those of people who, knowing that they are dying, face the fact frontally and act accordingly: They set their affairs in order, they arrange what could be final meetings with their loved ones, and yet, with strength of soul and a small reservoir of hope, they continue to live and love as much as they can for as long as they can. And, when the end finally draws nigh, they even "arrange" for the final parting, giving a lasting gift to those left behind.

My wife's mother, the proverbial woman of worth ("Her price is far above rubies"), left us such a legacy. Dying after a five-year struggle with breast cancer, riddled with painful bony metastases yet determined to take a proper leave, she returned home from the hospital and had my physician father-in-law summon all the children and grandchildren from across the country. She spoke privately to each of her children, telling my wife (gently, and without bitterness and self-pity), "When it is over, go and have a good cry and then get on with your life." She kept asking for her eldest son, coming from California, telling him "to hurry"—he did. Finally, with all assembled around her bed, she lay listening to a tape recording of the Friday evening Sabbath service, recorded for her by the cantor of her synagogue. In keeping with her character and lifelong habit, she gave not a hint of her own pains or sorrows. Precisely when the tape came to the end, with the final *Alenu* prayer that concludes all three daily services—finishing, in translation: "And it is said: 'The Lord will be King over all the earth, and on that day the Lord shall be One and His Name shall be One'"— she closed her eyes and died—serenely and beautifully. None of us present can think of this, her final gift, without smiling.

CAUTIONS AND QUESTIONS

There are, of course, several large asterisks that must be attached to all this uplifting talk about the possibility of living fully while being treated for cancer and about "dying well." First of all, medicine and life are, paradoxically, deeply at odds with each other, in theory and in practice. Modern medicine treats death as the enemy always to be opposed, disease as always to be cured, suffering as always to be relieved. Modern medicine is in principle opposed to finitude, and acts as if every death is a failure, to be cured by tomorrow's discoveries. In practice, this translates tragically into a necessary yet demoralizing medicalization of the very life it seeks to save and preserve. It treats people as patients (passive both to the disease and to the doctor's ministrations), not persons—for the doctors, my wife is a cancer patient, not a woman, teacher, wife, mother, and grandmother who happens, alas, also to have cancer.

For a person with cancer (and her family), the desire to concentrate on living her finite life to the full is undermined by being tethered to the chemotherapy parlor, by the necessity and frequency of treatment, and by the need always to attend to its often severe side effects. Weekly blood counts, daily booster injections, blood transfusions, the wearing of masks and the refusal of a grandchild's embrace for fear of infection, ointments for blisters, creams for cracking skin, hourly mouth washes for mouth sores, home monitoring of temperature and blood pressure, ice packs for burning hands and feet, pills for nausea or diarrhea or constipation—all these medically required attentions to one's diseased body and alterations of daily life get in the way of living—and of *thinking* and *feeling* about living—in anything like a normal way.

Even for a life-affirming and life-loving person such as my wife, little given to self-attention, it takes an extraordinary effort to keep the medicalization of her existence from eating away at the possibilities and enjoyments of her still largely vibrant life. How to negotiate the balance between these two perspectives on life—the life-preserving yet life-corroding view of medicine, and the vulnerable yet life-fulfilling view of ordinary existence—is perhaps the deepest and most subtle ethical task we face.

Edifying talk about living fully and dying well may also strike the reader as precious or as mere whistling in the dark, an attempt merely to make a virtue out of necessity—which I freely confess that it is, but adding in extenuation that much of human virtue is in fact born of necessity and the need to make something of it. Once again, it is likely that time will teach me more painful lessons, should my wife begin to suffer from her cancer and not only from its treatments.

Two of my colleagues in this volume have witnessed the bitter ends of their wonderful marriages, both of which came with agony and degradation for their beloveds. The desire and possibility of "making a good end of it" is, like life itself, not always or ever fully under our control. Few of us will be able to "engineer" or be given a humanized death-bed finale, let alone a death at home surrounded by children and grandchildren assembled to receive blessings and to say farewell. Yet, even as death now takes place on the doctor's watch—usually in the dehumanizing environment of hospitals in circumstances in which death receives no quarter or, better, in the humane setting of hospices where death is no longer treated as the enemy—there remain better and worse ways of going out and better and worse ways of accompanying life to its final exit.

For us spouses, there is always the complex but redemptive vocation of love, which both keeps company and respects solitude, to the very last moment of the story. Love recognizes that, as the old ballad has it, "You've got to cross that lonesome valley; you've got to cross it by yourself." When the time finally comes, it must be able to "give permission" for the lonely crossing to be made, and not burden the dying beloved with guilt for abandoning the surviving lover. Yet, at the same time, love steadfastly holds hands, rubs backs, and performs all the little—and large—offices of fidelity, loyalty, reliable presence, and loving affection. It knows that abandonment and withholding of support is betrayal, that presence and attachment are, especially in the ultimate hour, love's own highest office.

I have omitted two huge (and not unrelated) subjects that belong in the center of any discussion of ethics and mortality: the centrality of hope (and the problem of despair), and the question of life after death. In the belief of many people, even in our increasingly secular culture, death is not regarded as the end. Seeing the evils of earthly dying and loss as forerunners of a redeemed life hereafter carries also the more than consoling prospect of a heavenly reunion and takes at least a little of the sting out of the experienced agony of dying and parting. About the truth of all this, I remain agnostic—I will be pleasantly surprised if it is true, but I have never for a moment counted on it. And I confess to being both envious of the fortitude and horrified by the equanimity with which certain religious friends of mine accept the death of loved ones, even those who die very young leaving behind small children.

And yet, afterlife or no afterlife, I want to affirm the blessing and value of hope—by which I mean not optimism or what Arthur Frank has called "transitive hope," a hope *for* this or that *outcome*, but "intransitive hope," hope as a virtue, a way of holding oneself in life, a posture that can see, feel, and enact the possibility of goodness in the world, even when everything suggests that despair would be the more fitting attitude. Hope comes to us mysteriously, even in the darkness, and one does well and right by not refusing its offer. I hope (transitively) that I will be able to hold and display this blessed disposition when and if I really need it.

TOWARD AN ETHICS OF LIVING WITH MORTALITY

What, then, returning to the subject of this volume, can any of these experiences and reflections do for a richer bioethics? What generalizations, if any, can I offer for thinking about living with cancer, indeed, with living with mortality? Nothing at all, if one's penchant in ethics is to look for rules, guidelines, or public policies. But if ethics is the search for wisdom regarding "How to live?" perhaps some hints are possible, beginning with the call to attend seriously to the large existential questions.

A fertile—and helpful—field of bioethical examination should be opened up to consider the following subjects: how to defend both the idea and practice of living, immediately and wholeheartedly, against the corrosive inroads of medicalization; how to encourage a more realistic and shapely view of the life cycle, where the end of life is neither banished from the view of respectable opinion nor treated shallowly as a practical problem seeking technical solution; how to ensure that loving presence and fidelity are not casualties of the battle for longer life; how to help people learn to think about the *art* of living well—and dying well—in the face of mortal illness, not seduced by the techno- and bureaucratic "solutions" of "living wills" and annual discussions of end-of-life care with one's doctor; and how to think about the nature and meaning of hope, a virtue beyond optimism, that enables one to stand erect when the winds are howling and all that matters to you is in danger of being swept away.

Can bioethics do more? Beyond recommending that these subjects be restored to the center of ethical reflection, can we offer any ethical suggestions—even normative ethical suggestions—to persons with cancer and their loved ones? At first glance, it seems doubtful. How people speak and act in these difficult situations will vary greatly from person to person, depending on basic temperament, character, life experience, the presence or absence of engaging work and love, socio-economic circumstances, and the nature of the person's ultimate beliefs. That, after all, is what we learn most from the narrative approach to our subject. We can relate to other people's stories, yet we form our own according to our significantly different aspirations, attitudes, and attachments. No one, no matter how empathetic, can get inside another's skin, especially when it comes to suffering.

Yet, I also wonder if bioethics—or ethics more generally—might not have something normative to say to all this heterogeneity. I am, again, thinking not about rules or rights and wrongs, but about character, about those virtues of necessity that are especially needed in facing the ultimate necessity. Can we not find stories of fine character and fine conduct that can furnish the imagination and help shape hearts and minds? Can we not find examples to inspire—and others to avoid—that will make up for the lack of experience and point the way to admirable speech and deed? Should we not, in our search for wisdom, be consulting our rich religious traditions, as well as the writings of those poets, novelists, and philosophers, who, on whatever ground, believe that we human beings ought to be able to give an account for how we have lived—and helped others to live—within the realm of finitude?

Truth to tell, there is surely a limit to how much honest experience can be reconfigured and shaped by thinking, even the best thinking. Life is hard, and sometimes painful and grievous, and thought alone neither moves nor solves anything. Still, I have long been very impressed by two comments, neither of them from my own religious tradition, concerning desirable attitudes toward time and embodiment, attitudes that I have seen beautifully displayed even in the face of deadly disease.

St. Francis, in his garden planting onions, was asked what he would do were he to learn that he would die tomorrow. "Continue planting onions," was the answer. The implicit suggestion is that we should live each day in a way that matters, no matter how near or far our deaths. The second prescription (from St. Augustine): "Take care of your body as if you were going to live forever; and take care of your soul as if you were going to die tomorrow." The implicit suggestion is that we should treasure both the perishable body and the immortal soul, celebrating the mysterious concretion of the transient and the eternal that *is* our *human* being. Both these teachings, easy to applaud if hard to follow, might be said to be most appropriate for a thoughtful finite being, who appreciates the gift of bodily (hence finite) life, no matter how long our personal thread may be.

Does our secular culture (and secular bioethics), largely thoughtless about finitude and the life cycle, need something like the experience with cancer to reach the same insights? And, is there something that we (for-the-time-being) survivors and spouses of survivors can "teach," not just about life with cancer, but about living as such? It remains to be seen. But we can provide a proper beginning if we affirm and promote the need for such age-old wisdom.

Notes

1. Proverbs 31:25.
2. Psalms 90:12.
3. "The Case for Mortality," *The American Scholar* 52 (1983): 173–91. Reprinted (slightly revised) as "Mortality and Morality: The Virtues of Finitude" in my *Toward a More Natural Science: Biology and Human Affairs* (New York: The Free Press, 1985), 299–317, and (further revised) as "*L'Chaim* and Its Limits: Why Not Immortality?" in my *Life, Liberty, and the Defense of Dignity: The Challenge for Bioethics* (San Francisco: Encounter Books, 2002), 257–74. The point of departure of these essays was a set of futuristic proposals to treat death as just another disease and to try to conquer it entirely. The question, highly speculative, was whether human life would be better or worse off in the absence of mortality. The present point of departure, grounded in present reality, is the fact of a mortal illness that is attacking my beloved wife, life partner, and best friend. The questions we face are anything but speculative.
4. *Odyssey*, trans. Richmond Lattimore (New York: Harper & Row, 1965), V, 215–24.
5. Our report, *Taking Care: Ethical Caregiving in Our Aging Society*, was published in September, 2005. Retrieved February 11, 2011, from http://bioethics.georgetown.edu/pcbe/reports/taking_care/index.html
6. This, I venture to suggest, should be the ethical aspiration of living with this dread disease—easy to say, hard to realize.

CHAPTER 14

Survivorship

In Every Expression a Crack

Arthur W. Frank

I was treated for cancer in 1986–1987, and I began writing about my illness experiences in 1989.[1] I thus undertook a particularly public survivorship, including multiple speaking engagements in which I was billed on conference programs as a cancer survivor. I was not always what my hosts expected or wanted.

As pretentious as the comparison may be, I have identified with a section in the autobiography of Frederick Douglass, in which he describes being taken on speaking tours by the Abolitionists who supported him after he escaped from slavery. He is immensely grateful to these men, but he also resents their demand that he continue to be what audiences expected as an escaped slave, including "a *little* of the plantation manner of speech."[2] Douglass realizes his story might be new to each audience, "but it was the same old story to me," he writes. Acknowledging that these men were his friends and benefactors, and their advice was "not altogether wrong," Douglass concludes: "Still I must speak just the word that seemed to *me* the word to be spoken *by* me."

William Lloyd Garrison and others wanted Douglass simply to tell his story. But his story was no longer simple, "for I was now reading and thinking." Very soon after I finished treatment for cancer, I too was reading and thinking.

My problem, exemplified in what this chapter says and does not say, is that after a quarter century of reading and thinking about cancer, I am acutely aware that almost all of the words that I can speak are others' words. Often, what I once wrote no longer brings back embodied memories, but reads as one account among others; reading long-familiar stories of others' illnesses, I half remember their experiences as being my own. I am no longer certain what words ever were "spoken *by* me."

In the mid-1980s, being a survivor was more difficult in some ways than it is now, and in other ways it was easier. The difficulty was because there were still so many silences. After my treatments ended, I received multiple cues that cancer was supposed to be *over*. I recall poignant encounters with other survivors expressing the same problem. As one young woman put it, "No one wants me to talk about cancer, *but I have a lot more to say*." And yet, those silences also made being a survivor easier, because—and here I reach a major theme of this chapter—there were far fewer voices prescribing what cancer survivors should feel and do. Survivorship was just on the cusp of being commercialized—a provocative word that I will seek to justify—and if silence was isolating, it also allowed me to think about what had happened to me and discover my own language for expressing it.

Today, so many languages press themselves upon a cancer survivor, already filling silence in which words that could be called one's own might be discovered. Survivorship, as I will try to show, has become an industry, trading in expectations and self-images. The word *survivor* is itself contentious: embraced by some people who have had cancer as expressing how they imagine themselves, living in the shadow of an ordeal that they did survive; others simply accept *survivor* as the best available word; and some reject it because it implies a heroism they find false, suggesting some superiority of those who lived versus those who die.

Let me put these same thoughts another way, framing them between two quotations. The first has nothing to do with cancer but says everything about survivorship, at least as I have experienced it. The quotation is from the Russian philosopher and literary critic Mikhail Bakhtin, writing in the 1920s about Dostoevsky. "In every voice [Dostoevsky] could hear two contending voices," Bakhtin writes, "*in every expression a crack*, and the readiness to go over immediately to another contradictory expression" (emphases added).[3]

Twenty-five years after cancer, that passage is how I imagine survivorship. My voice was always cracked: confident that I could write as a survivor, but lacking confidence in my survival; grateful to my physicians and nurses, to my family and loved ones, to my friends, to my colleagues and employer, but also resenting things they did or left undone; feeling that, for me, cancer carried a sense of responsibility, but reluctant to assert that as a duty for all survivors. What has filled that crack, and still fills it after all these years, are other voices. My voice has always been contending voices, one always about to give way to another.

Bakhtin's evocative phrase, "in every expression a crack," is exemplified by another voice of illness. "I now realize that I will never have a single conclusion about my cancer," wrote Fitzhugh Mullan in his memoir, *Vital Signs*. "Perhaps it was naïve to have ever thought that I would."

> Even as I write about it I can feel a kind of terminal ambivalence about the entire experience. Though I would never have chosen to have cancer, it is part of me and therefore something that I can't hate, deny, or discard. Like a lame leg or a blind eye, it is with me for the rest of my life. For better *and* for worse, I will live with it and quietly work and rework my personal history in an effort to accommodate it as much as possible.[4]

When I first read this passage, probably in 1992 or '93, I felt ambivalent about Mullan's ambivalence. At that point in the trajectory of my survival of cancer, I wanted a more definitive statement. Rereading Mullan today, he speaks to me, and for me, with perfect accuracy. I have become capable of claiming my own ambivalence and can only wonder that it took me so long.

To write about survivorship, then, I can only recall the voices that have meant the most to me. I agree with what Rebecca Dresser writes in Chapter 1, that all of us are wondering what to make of our personal experiences with cancer. But, having lived with those experiences for much longer than the other group members, my experiences now come back to me in others' voices, especially voices I have written about. Some of these voices sound old, in the sense of dated. Others remind me of forgotten wisdom, and I ask myself whether I have grown deaf to what I could once hear. As this chapter moves to contemporary voices, I hear them less as a fellow-sufferer who seeks—sometimes desperately—for words to express what I felt but could not articulate. Instead, I hear contemporary voices as an observer of strangers whose problems are recognizable but no longer mine. And yet, I know how immediately that could change, because one thing I have not forgotten is the terrible suddenness with which illness transforms a life. And that recognition of how utterly different words might sound tomorrow is another crack.

VOICES OF SURVIVORSHIP

During the first decade after my treatment for cancer, four voices stand out as loudest in the chorus of multiple voices that has become my voice. The first, both in chronology and in pride of place, is the activist voice of the poet Audre Lorde, who claimed survivorship within what I would now call identity politics. I use that term to describe advocacy (politics in the most generic sense) based on the privilege of experiential voices and their capacity to speak the truth of institutions and their priorities, such as health care.[5] Lorde's work encouraged me to think of survivorship as a political project of making cancer visible and gaining recognition for what society marginalized. In her writing, there is none of Mullan's ambivalence. The message is clear: Make connections with other ill people and demand recognition.

Lorde imagines—as much as anyone, she invents—*survivorship* as the self-conscious shaping of identity and its projects to address what cancer asks and even requires of the political individual. The project of survivorship begins with what Lorde calls "my right to define and to claim my own body."[6] Lorde's telling of her own story is punctuated by diverse "assaults" on this right. Some of these are benign, such as the visit from a Reach for Recovery volunteer whose heterosexual assumptions amuse Lorde (who is gay), but also leave her feeling estranged from culturally dominant understandings of cancer and survival. Lorde becomes angry at institutional medicine as it fronts the prosthetic demands of society: Medicine *works* to sustain the invisibility of illnesses like breast cancer. For her, public appearance as one-breasted is an essential act of witness and solidarity.

In the issue of visibility, the personal is political: Prostheses seek to render cancer invisible, and thus they make any community of cancer survivors impossible. "It is very difficult sometimes to remember that I AM NOT ALONE," Lorde writes. "Yet, once I face death as a life process, what is there possibly left for me to fear? Who can ever really have power over me again?"[7] When I first read these words, they enabled me to acknowledge how utterly alone I had felt during cancer, despite the kindest attention of my wife, family, and friends, as well as what in retrospect seems excellent medical treatment (a judgment that may say more about how my expectations for medicine have softened). Survivorship was finding ways out of that aloneness and fear, and Lorde's blunt statement—in capital letters—was an enormous relief.

Reading Lorde twenty years ago, her writing spoke to the sense of stigma I still remembered not only vividly but viscerally, when I began to tell people I might have cancer and the fear that my presence generated while I was visibly in treatment. During the year before my cancer diagnosis, I had a virally induced heart attack, and I had just left cardiac care when I reported symptoms of cancer to my physician. I was acutely aware of how different I felt telling people I had cancer, as opposed to giving news of my heart problems, and I was aware of how differently people reacted. The stigma of cancer was unmistakable. Lorde also spoke to my sense of suspicion about medicine. I went through a long period of misdiagnosis, during which I was in extraordinary pain; this left me highly suspicious of medicine.

Finally, although there is no particular end to her influence on me, Lorde reinforced my developing understanding of cancer as a problem of communication and testimony. A decade earlier, I had written my doctoral dissertation on personal accounts of death and dying, some by dying persons themselves but most by spouses and adult children. Even though published memoirs of illness did not yet constitute a recognizable genre, I was definitely aware of such memoirs during my own illnesses. I always thought of cancer as creating a need to speak and an imperative to learn. "I had known the pain, and survived it," Lorde wrote. "It only remained for me to give it voice, to share it for use, that the pain not be wasted."[8] I read those words after I had written my own book, but while I was still uncertain where survivorship went from there. She affirmed my sense that I had only begun the journey.

As important as Audre Lorde was to me, the voice of the identity politics of survivorship that most clearly spoke to the work of writing and public speaking that I was undertaking was a woman given the pseudonym of Gail, interviewed by the anthropologist Linda Garro as part of a project on chronic pain. Gail expresses the divides on which an identity politics of survivorship is based. She is divided from the healthy, including medical professionals, by both her distinct knowledge, and by the embodiment that enables that knowledge.

> And all these people in pain . . . all these people with aches and all these people suffering. We walk in different dimensions. We have access to different knowledges. And there are so many of us, too. What would happen if we all knew what it really meant and we all lived as if it really mattered, which it does. We could help the normals and the whitecoats both. We could help them see that they're wasting the precious moments of their lives, if they would look at us who don't have it. I'm convinced only sick people know what health is. And they know it by its very loss.[9]

Through the mid-1990s, Gail's voice summarized for me both the ethical demand of survivorship and also what being a survivor made possible. To have cancer is to have access to a form of knowledge that others lack; that knowledge matters, and there is a responsibility to convey it.

Gail's claim to knowledge underpins the project of which this book is part. The issue is not so much whether we who have lived through cancer have access to knowledge that other bioethicists lack—of course we do, but then everyone has certain knowledge that others lack. A better phrasing might be to ask what sort of issues in bioethics might be responded to differently, if the response was informed by experiential knowledge. Bioethics is a very big tent, but in most parts of it, Gail's claim would not elicit much interest; professional competence in bioethics is not understood to depend on personal experience. Indeed, claims to privileged knowledge based on personal experience can be threatening to professional competence, in bioethics as in other spheres of expertise.

A very different and more generalized call to lead an *active* survivorship came from the writing of Albert Schweitzer, who was the iconic figure of Christian commitment and winner of the Nobel Peace Prize when I was growing up in the 1950s. Schweitzer's first medical mission to Africa was ended by World War I, and he was interned by the French as an enemy alien. The conditions of internment were respectful, but the privations led to acute illness requiring a sequence of surgeries. As he recovered from his own illness, Schweitzer reconceived his missionary work as the personal responsibility of one who had known suffering to aid those who now suffer. When I quoted Schweitzer in my 1995 study of illness narratives, *The Wounded Storyteller*, the quotation was a direct expression of my own attitude toward survivorship:

> Whoever among us has learned through personal experience what pain and anxiety really are must help to ensure that those out there who are in physical need obtain the same help that once came to him. He no longer belongs to himself alone; he has become the brother of all who suffer. It is this "brotherhood of those who bear the mark of pain" that demands humane medical services.[10]

Schweitzer expresses most directly the idea of survivorship as moral responsibility. I recall flying back to Calgary one night after a speaking engagement and by chance sitting next to someone I knew. I was talking about my life and survivorship activities, and he said to me, "It's cost you a great deal to do what you're doing." I heard his tone to be intended as half caution and half criticism. He spoke from the counseling perspective that is expressed in phrases like "getting on with your life." He recognized that, in order to do the writing and speaking that were my work, I had to keep part of myself ill, and that had real costs. But I took his words as a kind of blessing. Survivorship, in the Schweitzer version, is supposed to have a cost. Nothing less is expected.

Schweitzer appealed to me, in part, because of the spiritual resonances in his writing. Cancer, for me, had been marked by several spiritual experiences that were intense enough at the time, but intensified further as I reworked them in what I wrote.[11] This spiritual voice had multiple sources, but the one that now is most audible to me is my own. In *At the Will of the Body*, I describe an afternoon during chemotherapy when I saw, as if for the first time, a framed poster of Marc Chagall's stained-glass window of Jacob wrestling with the angel. Staring at that picture—entering it—I felt a deep identification with that story:

> Stories come to us from many sources; some we seek, many happen to us without our notice, others impose themselves on our lives. We have to choose carefully which stories to live with, which to use to answer the question of what is happening to us. Jacob's wrestling became a story I lived with as part of my personal mythology of illness. That is what it is to be ill: to wrestle through the long night, injured, and if you prevail until the sun rises, to receive a blessing.[12]

That voice, today, I surely recognize as my own. In that voice I was creating the terms of my survivorship by telling what was, quite literally, a story I could live with. But here again, my story is nine-tenths borrowed story.

Certainly in retrospect, my survivorship has been a process of constantly sifting and reformulating what counts as experience: what will be remembered, how it will be told, and what it will be connected to. My own experience differs, perhaps, from that of many cancer survivors in that, because I was doing this sifting and reformulating in print, there is a trail I can follow. I hear the voices along that trail as one greets an old friend: certainly recognizing him, but a bit wary of how we may have grown apart. That wariness is part of my current affinity to the ambivalence expressed by Mullan.

NOISY SURVIVORSHIP

Flash forward twenty-plus years to today, not so many years later but a very different time to be a cancer survivor. A recent story in Toronto's

Globe and Mail newspaper profiles two women whose survival is apparently due to the drug Herceptin. The story is about their struggles to get funding for treatment with Herceptin, but a good deal else is said about the nature of survivorship. The fact that major newspapers regularly run full-page feature stories on cancer and survivorship is one measure of how much things have changed since Audre Lorde challenged people living with cancer to cease being silent. Today, survivorship is highly visible, and the individual problem is figuring out in which terms to participate. Nonparticipation seems less and less optional, as the *Globe* story suggests.

The *Globe* story focuses on Nathalie Le Prohon, formerly president of Nokia Canada, diagnosed with breast cancer in 2004. The story frames Ms. Le Prohon in a rhetoric of heroic achievement: "For Nathalie Le Prohon, the one lesson she can impart from the Herceptin campaign is that patients must be their own advocates. 'I truly believe I am alive because of all this. . . I was always an extremely busy, career woman who gets results. So I attacked the cancer the same way.'"[13]

The article then describes how Ms. Le Prohon paid privately to receive Herceptin in the United States before it was available in Canada, and finally got access at home when Herceptin was approved in Ontario. Her subsequent survivorship is presented as an extension of her business career, almost a caricature of hyperactivity: "Today, her life is focused on advocacy rather than swinging big business deals: She does charity runs, fundraises for children's schools and is chair of the Quebec Breast Cancer Foundation, and has considered running as a Liberal candidate for parliament." Yet, the narrative is not entirely heroic. Ms. Le Prohon is also quoted as saying: "Every time I go for a new mammogram, the worry creeps in again. You have to live with that all your life. You are never cancer free. You are always thinking: 'When will the beast return?'"

The newspaper account depicts survivorship within a network of business, finance (cost of medications and distribution of that cost), politics (lobbying for access), medical knowledge, and emotion work ("the worry"). The phrase that is most striking to me, contrasting this account with what could have been said or thought in the 1980s, is how Herceptin "helped Ms. Le Prohon make the best of her cancer experience." As a phrase in public discourse, *making the best* is resonant with codes of consumerism as well as self-help and self-improvement.[14] *Her cancer experience* is resonant with such phrases as *vacation experience*, *dining experience*, or in my own field, *education experience*. Survivorship is thus *being positioned* by the article, which is what journalism necessarily does: Stories like this one position identities within discourses (finance, medical, self-help and so on) and their respective codes of interpretation; mass media articles create self-images and the expectations that go with them. To its credit, this article then presents a very different positioning of survivorship.

The *Globe* article continues by introducing Leslie Cowan, who also seems to be alive because of Herceptin, but who tells a very different survivorship story. Ms. Cowan's profile begins with a preface that reflects on the public discourse of cancer survivorship, a discourse in which the article itself is participating—an inescapable loop.

> Cancer does not end when treatment does, yet a public bombarded by inspirational stories has expectations of what a survivor should be.
>
> At age 40, Leslie Cowan was diagnosed with stage-3C cancer—the nearest curable step to the fatal stage 4. The culprit was a tumour roughly the size of an apricot. [Earlier in the article, Ms. Le Prohon's tumour is equated to a "quail egg"]. . . .
>
> With her treatment behind her, Ms. Cowan says she no longer looks like a cancer patient—but she still sometimes feels like one. "What I find is when you're bald or you look sick, people are great, they bring you dinner," she says. "The minute you start to look good, people think, 'You're fine.' That's when you need the support the most. And there's nowhere to go."[15]

So far, Ms. Cowan's story could have been written during the 1980s, except that such stories did not appear then. But her complaint is what members of 1980s support groups then talked about: If people with cancer were marginalized, cancer survivors were completely invisible. But then Ms. Cowan's story moves in directions that were barely imaginable in the 1980s:

> She became obsessed for a time with making the most of her reprieve from death, perhaps by climbing a mountain or working in an orphanage in a developing country. [Ms. Cowan has two children.]
>
> "I feel like I failed Cancer 101. I got one shot at it. I didn't climb Kilimanjaro. I haven't written a book," says Ms. Cowan, who used to work in fundraising and public relations. "There's this pressure to do something spectacular with your life because you have cancer. It didn't result in some greater meaning for me."
>
> It's hard to escape these expectations. Each October, in Breast Cancer Awareness Month, an avalanche of pink products hits shelves— ribbons, hats, T-shirts and blenders. Inspirational stories fill papers and magazines.

For Ms. Cowan, there was fallout: Her marriage faltered and she sought the help of a psychiatrist . . . .

"I don't know why I feel I need to give back to something that took so much. I don't care how many people say it made their life better. I don't believe that."

The article goes on to discuss "the icon of the cancer super-hero" and the stress that image can create. If Ms. Le Prohon is a somewhat qualified "cancer super-hero," Ms. Cowan balances that by being a credible and sympathetic anti-hero. Her story expresses resistance to what were originally resistances. Her voice is filled with voices she may never have heard, including my own. But while my problem of survivorship was breaking out of silence, hers may be finding a still point amid all the noise. This problem could have been anticipated.

PUBLIC SURVIVORSHIP AND ITS CONTROVERSIES

In the early 1990s, colleagues, especially in Britain where personal accounts of illness were published less often, cautioned me that the version of survivorship I was advocating—based on voices like Audre Lorde, Gail, and Albert Schweitzer—could result in expectations that some people would find oppressive. For me, that danger was outweighed by the need to create multiple possibilities for people to express themselves in response to cancer. Critics, I felt, had simply not heard what Audre Lorde and Gail were saying so eloquently. The crucial difference seemed to be between an empowered sense of what someone who had cancer *could* do and a disempowering sense of what survivors were *expected* to do. There was virtually no public discourse of survivorship as possibility, and creating that discourse seemed to have priority. Such a public discourse has emerged, but not as Audre Lorde imagined it.

In the 1990s, the publication of many first-person narratives of cancer, including my own, was probably less important than the shift in patient support services from the older model exemplified by Reach to Recovery, with its goal of the former patient achieving invisibility, to newer models of public survivorship, exemplified by participation in civic fitness events for survivors—and wearing the tee shirt afterward. The flip point of reaction against those public models was the publication of Barbara Ehrenreich's "Welcome to Cancerland" article in 2001,[16] with its withering description of how women are not empowered but are infantilized by the avalanche of pink products.

The Women's Studies scholar Samantha King extends Ehrenreich's critique in her study of how breast cancer became the optimal site for corporate philanthropy and how corporate influence has changed survivorship. King summarizes what has changed since Audre Lorde asked, "What would happen if an army of one-breasted women descended upon Congress and demanded that the use of carcinogenic, fat-stored hormones in beef-feed be outlawed?"[17] King points out that the army of one-breasted women now *does* assemble in Washington, but they participate in a fundraising run, and corporations are the sponsors, not the objects of protest. Participation is not just athletic; the events also *position* survivors with respect to appropriate expectations and actions.

> In certain respects, then, Lorde's vision has been realized: breast cancer is rarely viewed now as a shameful or self-induced disease and is . . . most often portrayed as an enriching and affirming experience during which women with breast cancer are rarely categorized as "victims" or "patients.". . . But Lorde's warning that to look on the bright side of things is to obscure realities that might prove threatening to the dominant order is more relevant now than ever before.
>
> While it is quite common for illness to function as a transformative experience on an individual basis, often in positive ways, the dominant discourse of breast cancer survivorship . . . leaves little room for alternative, less positive, understandings of the disease experience and its long-term effects, or relatedly, of the political-economic context in which the fight against the disease is being waged.[18]

Although Audre Lorde argued the desirability of particular choices for some women—most notably, the rejection of prostheses—her overall position is to affirm the primacy of choice itself; for example, "Every woman has a right to define her own desires, make her own choices."[19] Her argument against prostheses begins with them not being chosen.

King's argument is that since Lorde, "One individualizing narrative has thus been replaced by another."

> The new narrative of individual responsibility allows women to get sick but not to die and, in circulating the ideal model of survivorship, succeeds in selling an enormous range of goods to consumers, raising millions of dollars for large nonprofits [and, King demonstrates, for their corporate partners], and garnering votes for politicians eager to find an issue that positions them as prowoman but not feminist. The model also helps to maintain support for high-stakes, early detection,

and cure-oriented research to the virtual exclusion of other avenues of exploration.[20]

King's argument explains why, several years ago, I donated my considerable number of health charity tee shirts to a clothing donation bin. Once it seemed like wearing them was a response to Lorde's call for the visibility of cancer survivors. As the survivorship industry intensified, I felt like a walking billboard, providing free advertising for corporate entities, including the charity itself. My reaction remains ambivalent. I respect the work done by groups dedicated to improving survivorship, but it seems to me that the quality of that work is inverse to the size of the group: smaller is better. Funding is a constant struggle for small groups, but the lack of corporate ties—and not being a corporate entity themselves—offers these groups a freedom of expression that is lost as the number of "partnerships" increases. As King so convincingly demonstrates, each of those partners expects something in return for their support, and that shapes the public image of survivorship.

CONCLUDING AMBIVALENCES

It's a long way from *At the Will of the Body* to *Pink Ribbons, Inc.* I am glad that my work written in the 1980s remains in print and that it seems to meet a need among people living with cancer and other illnesses. But while my task then was to enable a new language of survivorship, what I think is needed today are critiques of a corporatized jargon of survivorship that people like Leslie Cowan and Barbara Ehrenreich experience as an imposition, requiring a particular response to cancer. What can be made of it all?

First, survivorship takes place at a certain time, in a certain place, and in that time and place, some narratives and discourses will be dominant, others will be oppositional, and still others will be unspoken, waiting for someone to give them voice. Who people are able to be and how they live with cancer depends on the narrative resources that these discourses make available. When I had cancer, there seemed to be far too few narrative resources available. Today, people with cancer seem assailed by narratives that compete to represent their experiences and set their future agendas.

Second, with respect to what cancer survivors might do or be expected to do: *People are called differently* in survivorship. As I wrote earlier, the line between possibility and expectation may be a fine one, but it is crucial to observe that line. When I read Ms. Cowan's line that she hadn't written a book about having cancer, I thought she must be joking. It took me a moment to realize that she meant this seriously and spoke with a sense of deficiency. That she feels this way is immensely sad, to say the least.

Third, what is struggled for in one decade may need to be opposed in the next. Personal struggles *of* survivorship have always reflected collective struggles *for* survivorship; that is, the struggle to define what is valued as a personal and as a collective response to illness. Audre Lorde felt she was battling to make cancer visible. Today, breast cancer especially is highly visible, but *what* has been made visible is worth questioning. Once, it took considerable fortitude just to say the C-word. Today, the omnipresence of publicity about cancer—heroic survivors and prospective cures—conceals continuing silences about differential access to treatment, especially in the United States, and lack of precaution with respect to possible environmental causes of cancer, among other issues.

Fourth, if these struggles have changed during my own survivorship, it is that more codes are now invoked, with increasing financial stakes on the primacy of particular codes. The survivor has become a marketing target, and anticorporate groups are equally anxious to enroll her. Survivorship, then, is a site of contest between diverse discourses. The question for any survivor is how well you can reflectively understand which discourses you embody, and then, which do you choose to embody, insofar as it is possible to speak of *choice*.[21]

In conclusion, but not conclusively, to be a cancer survivor long enough may doom a person to ambivalence; one becomes, as Bakhtin says of Dostoevsky's characters, always ready "to go over immediately to another contradictory expression."[22] Or, to quote the stock punch line of a justly honored cancer survivor, Gilda Radner, "it's always something."[23] In response to any assertion about cancer survivorship, there will be a counterassertion. And, most often, each will address some real need. Like everyone, I live with the multiple voices in my head: some the voices of others, and some my own voices from earlier decades; some voices in harmony, others quarreling.

But I do come back to Gail, whose voice still sounds the clearest. All that has happened to me—what in retrospect was the very short period of having cancer and the many more years of being a survivor—has endowed me with what Gail called "access to different knowledges."[24] It's just that those knowledges are not the same knowledges I had when my scars had not yet faded. To return to Frederick Douglass's phrase, I have gone on reading and thinking.

I believe, as I did then, that things happen to us humans for absolutely no reason at all—a hair's width often separates disaster from triumph—but the gift of being human is our capacity to fill in the blanks: to transform chaos into narrative. My particular chaos could have been war or any number of other human misfortunes. It happened to be illness. A further gift of being human is our capacity to discriminate among stories; to decide which stories are better to live with than others, even if we never make those decisions in conditions of our own choosing. People can tell cancer stories any number of different ways, and in response to each of these, it's always something. But that doesn't mean we can stop working to tell the story that our time and place seems to call for.

Notes

1. Arthur W. Frank, *At the Will of the Body: Reflections on Illness* (Boston: Houghton Mifflin, 1991). The book was translated into German, Dutch, Spanish, and Japanese. In 2002, a new edition appeared under the Mariner Books imprint of the original publisher. The book remains distinctive insofar as it is one of the few illness memoirs written by someone who was not a previously published author, celebrity, or physician. I am also one of the very few authors (I know of four, including myself) of an illness memoir who has written subsequent nonmemoirs about illness and health care.
2. Frederick Douglass, *Autobiographies* (New York: Library of America, 1994), 367.
3. Mikhail Bakhtin, *Problems of Dostoevsky's Poetics*. Translated by Caryl Emerson (Minneapolis: University of Minnesota Press, 1984), 30.
4. Fitzhugh Mullan, *Vital Signs: A Young Doctor's Struggle With Cancer* (New York: Laurel, 1984), 195.
5. *Identity politics* has different meanings in different speech genres and is controversial. It has often been used as a term of deprecation; I myself have sometimes understood it as a put-down. Today, in 2010, I think it may be possible to use the term as a neutral description of the assumptions underpinning an advocacy stance. If that neutrality is possible, it may be because *identity politics* is dated, even worn out, as a phrase.
6. Audre Lorde, *The Cancer Journals* (San Francisco: spinsters/aunt lute, 1980), 59.
7. Lorde, *The Cancer Journals*, 61.
8. Lorde, *The Cancer Journals*, 16.
9. Quoted in Linda Garro, "Chronic Illness and the Construction of Narratives," in *Pain as Human Experience*, ed. Mary-Jo Delvecchio Good, Paul E. Brodwin, Byron J. Good, and Arthur Kleinman (Berkeley and Los Angeles: University of California Press, 1992), 129. See my use of this quotation in Arthur W. Frank, *The Wounded Storyteller: Body, Illness, and Ethics* (Chicago: University of Chicago Press, 1995), 141.

10. Quoted in Frank, *The Wounded Storyteller*, 35. The quotation is reprinted in numerous editions of Schweitzer's writing; my source was Schweitzer's autobiography, *Out of My Life and Thought*. Translated by Antje Bultman Lemke (1933; New York: Henry Holt, 1990), 195.

11. During the 1990s, I wrote review essays for *The Christian Century*, emphasizing spiritual responses to illness and issues of bioethics. I was also editor of a series of first-person illness stories in the journal *Second Opinion*, sponsored by The Park Ridge Center in Chicago, funded by the Lutheran Church. I continue to speak regularly at conferences on spiritual care.

12. Frank, *At the Will of the Body*, 81.

13. Lisa Priest, "A Wonder Drug, but Not a Miracle." *The Globe and Mail*, March 27, 2010, F5.

14. For relevant cultural history, see Anne Harrington, *The Cure Within: A History of Mind-Body Medicine* (New York: Norton, 2008), especially Chapter 3, "The Power of Positive Thinking." Although the *Globe* article situates cancer survivorship within biomedicine, aspects of the narrative of positive thinking inescapably enter its discourse.

15. Priest, "A Wonder Drug," F5.

16. Barbara Ehrenreich, "Welcome to Cancerland," *Harper's*, November 2001, 43–53.

17. Lorde, *The Cancer Journals*, 16.

18. Samantha King, *Pink Ribbons, Inc. Breast Cancer and the Politics of Philanthropy* (Minneapolis: University of Minnesota Press, 2006), 102. King's argument bears directly on issues raised in my chapter on support groups in this volume. Such groups assert the preferred identities of members as much by omission as by outright positive assertion.

19. Lorde, *The Cancer Journals*, 65.

20. King, *Pink Ribbons, Inc.*, 104.

21. The idea, and often the reification, of *choice* as a kind of solution to ethical problems is discussed in Annemarie Mol, *The Logic of Choice: Health and the Problem of Patient Choice* (London: Routledge, 2008).

22. Quoted earlier, n. 3.

23. Gilda Radner, *It's Always Something* (New York: Avon Books, 1990).

24. Quoted above, n. 10.

CHAPTER 15

Last Words

Rebecca Dresser

Cancer experiences resist simple analysis. If this book illuminates anything, it is the absence of a single take-home message about cancer. Yes, there are themes and shared judgments, and we report them in these pages. But there is individuality in cancer, too. In our individual contributions, each of us tells a particular story and interprets that story through a particular lens. In this chapter, I say a bit about each of our contributions, then move to broader themes. I explain why work like ours belongs in medical ethics—what it adds and why it is important. I close with thoughts on how cancer changed our perspectives on work and on life.

Norman Fost's commitment to good and fair medical practice is the foundation of his chapter on diagnosis. Norm's kidney cancer was diagnosed at a treatable stage because an emergency room doctor ordered a medically unnecessary scan. If Norm hadn't had the scan, he might not be alive today. Norm nevertheless insists that it is unethical to spend limited health care dollars on unwarranted interventions like the scan he received. He wants the health care system to change, so that privileged individuals like him don't receive the expensive, unjustified tests that every so often reveal cancer. The benefit he obtained from the unnecessary scan was immense, but it was unfair that he obtained it.

Norm also writes as a contrarian, taking a stance against mainstream perceptions of cancer. In our chapter on cancer stereotypes, Norm argues that cancer isn't always all it's cracked up to be. His own case shows that assumptions about cancer don't always hold true. Cancer doesn't necessarily deserve its status as the most frightening disease, for other diseases can be more menacing than cancer. It would be better for everyone if people paid more attention to the facts behind the terrifying label. In cancer, as in every serious illness, medical specifics and personal circumstances are what really matter. Cancer is a bad disease, but it should not eclipse the many other illnesses that can be just as devastating, and just as worthy of our moral concern.

John Robertson's chapters exhibit the law professor's concern for detail, but they are primarily the testimony of a grieving husband. John's stories are immediate, vivid, and revealing. Neither holding back, nor escaping into academic analysis, he exposes the raw emotions that continue to frame his cancer experience. John is also open about behavior he isn't proud of. What we learn from John's accounts is that he was a good and steadfast caregiver, not a saint. He was far from alone in his imperfection. Everyone in our group pleaded guilty to less-than-admirable conduct while dealing with cancer. People handle cancer as best they can, sometimes well, sometimes not so well.

John also writes about his wife Carlota's reluctance to engage in death talk, and his attempt to get her to confront the "elephant in the room." He reminds us that loved ones don't always deal with dying in the way that we expect them to, or want them to. For Carlota, awareness of mortality was one thing, mucking around in it was quite another. No one should force a patient to enter what is truly frightening territory; it would have been selfish to insist that she speak openly of her impending death. John was wise and compassionate in letting Carlota die in her own way, though he might have wished for something different.

In his chapters, Dan Brock writes as an analytic philosopher examining two classic topics in medical ethics: patient decision-making and allocation of health care resources. But Dan also writes as a cancer patient who discovered that philosophical analysis doesn't take into account the complexity of real-life medical decision-making. When he was diagnosed with prostate cancer, Dan assumed the role of the model autonomous patient. He regarded his illness as a problem to be solved, and he set about solving it. He searched the Internet, talked with many doctors, and consulted men who had been treated for prostate cancer. He came away with a wealth of information, but without a clear answer. He realized he needed something more—guidance from his doctor. He decided to have the surgery his doctor recommended, but was left with side effects he wasn't prepared for. Neither the doctors nor any other source had supplied the kind of information he needed to make his decision. Despite his extensive research, his consent was based on inadequate information.

Modern medicine is biased in favor of intervention, and patients often share this bias. In making his treatment choice, Dan discovered his own interventionist bias. Acknowledging his need to "do something" about his cancer, he admits to collaborating in the decision to go forward with the surgery that left him with serious side effects. Although watchful waiting would have been a rational and possibly more cost-effective option for him, Dan admits that he would not have been satisfied with that option. And, although he's convinced it would be ethical to restrict access to questionable-benefit cancer treatments, he confesses that he might resist such a rule if he encountered it as a patient. Dan is refreshingly candid about his discovery that the philosopher's view of ethical issues can be simplistic and incomplete.

My own stories are about classic medical ethics topics, too: treatment refusal and research participation. And, like Dan's chapters, they uncover problems often overlooked in standard ethics analysis. Although I was an informed and educated patient, I was vulnerable to irrational thinking that for a time led me to refuse an intervention I needed. I wanted desperately to survive, but I resisted the feeding tube that could help me reach this goal. My experience shows that patients who appear capable and qualified to make their own choices aren't always equipped to make good ones. As a seriously ill patient, I learned that exercising my decision-making authority was more difficult than I had anticipated.

I also describe what personal experience taught me about clinical trials. I saw first-hand the conflict between the doctor's duty to recommend the best treatment for his patient and the clinical researcher's duty to advance knowledge. And I learned how serious illness can affect a patient's judgments about trial enrollment. Facing a life-threatening cancer, I chose the treatment that seemed to offer me the greatest chance of survival. I was willing to make some contributions to the research effort, but I rejected a treatment trial that seemed to ask too much of me. Seriously ill people want—and are owed—good therapeutic alternatives. Researchers should do all they can to ensure that cancer trials offer patients not only reasonable risks, but also up-to-date treatment options.

In her chapters, Patricia Marshall reflects on her two cancer catastrophes. The first came when she was diagnosed with breast cancer and went through a long and difficult treatment regimen: two surgeries, chemotherapy, and radiation treatment. Not long after that, her husband Larry died of an aggressive and untreatable cancer. In "Resilience: The Art of Living in Remission," Patty describes the long and rocky road she has traveled since these two assaults. Although she has had a few years to recover from the acute crises, she still lives with their aftereffects. Every day, she sees and feels cancer's physical effects. Cancer's psychic effects are also inescapable. Each follow-up visit and test is unsettling, for someone might discover that she has cancer again. And now there is the terrifying prospect of facing cancer alone. Yet, Patty is resilient. In the face of these terrors, she moves forward, more fragile than she once was, yet still capable of joy and hope.

In our chapter on cancer interactions, Patty and I describe the astounding, the magnificent, and the appalling behavior we encountered when we were dealing with cancer. There is more than a little anger in some of our remarks. No doubt we were naïve about such matters before cancer entered our lives, but some of the behavior we witnessed left us speechless, and some of it left us fuming. Yet, we also encountered unexpected generosity. Cancer would have been much worse without the help of the many relatives, friends, and others who reached out to us. It may be frightening when someone you know gets cancer, but that is no excuse for insensitivity. It's possible to provide real comfort to people dealing with cancer, and we give examples of how this can be done.

Arthur Frank, the sociologist, writes about cancer interactions too, but with a different focus. His chapters describe the resources patients draw on to make sense of life during and after cancer. Art examines several cancer narratives available to patients, exposing the good and bad sides of each. As he points out, those controlling the narratives, such as support group leaders and corporate-sponsored charities, have their own interests and agendas. Art gives a compelling account of how other patients' voices helped him to forge his own post-cancer identity. Although he believes patients have an urgent need for narrative resources, he warns against relying too much on today's images and icons of cancer.

For Art, unlike the rest of us, cancer is an event in the distant past. It is also an event that transformed the life that came after. Making sense of having cancer, and of surviving it, became Art's personal and professional calling. It is a continuing pursuit, one characterized by instability and ambivalence—"in every expression a crack." And there are more twists and turns to come. Although it has been more than twenty years since his cancer treatment, Art remains painfully aware that a new threat could arise at any time. This long-term survivor will never forget "the terrible suddenness with which illness transforms a life."

Cancer refuses to grant many patients the long-lasting reprieve that Art has enjoyed. Treatment gave Leon Kass and his beloved wife a blissful period in which they "dared to hope" that her cancer was gone. But this was not to be. In his chapter on cancer and mortality, Leon offers an honest, heartfelt, and poignant account of how they are living, and trying to live, in the presence of what is now a metastatic cancer. Leon's sorrow is palpable—his reflections are moving and painful to read. He does not hold back in portraying cancer's miseries and evils; he is able to see it for what it is. Yet, he can also move beyond the bleakness to savor the love and life that remain. Leon asks the "big questions," the ones that come to the forefront when you are face-to-face with mortality.

Our chapters offer a variety of views on cancer. Each of us writes from a particular perspective, reflecting the specific cancers we dealt with, as well as our individual outlooks and professional backgrounds. And, although cancer is still a presence in all of our lives, it is a bigger presence in some lives than in others. On many matters, however, we speak with one voice. In our meeting discussions, as well as in our writing, we discovered much common ground. I turn now to that common ground.

WHY IS OUR BOOK A MEDICAL ETHICS BOOK?

Readers, including our medical ethics colleagues, might wonder how this book fits into medical ethics. The things we write about may be important to sick people and to their families and doctors, but why are they relevant to medical ethics?[1] Aren't we simply discussing patient care and the experience of serious illness?

The relationship between patients and doctors has always been at the heart of medical ethics. Beginning with the Hippocratic Oath, medical ethics pledges and codes have been most concerned with the way doctors behave toward their patients. And in the 1970s, when medical ethics entered the public arena, the focus remained on the doctor–patient relationship. The death-with-dignity and patients' rights movements emerged because people were worried about what doctors might do to them if they became seriously ill. They wanted some control over their treatment, and they wanted information about their treatment options. But not all doctors were willing to relinquish their customary power over patients' care. And even doctors committed to sharing power were unsure how to do it. Medical schools and hospitals turned to ethics for help in thinking through the issues raised by this new vision of clinical care. Most of us went into the medical ethics field because we found these matters both fascinating and significant.

Since the 1970s, however, the medical ethics field has become much broader than it used to be. Now referred to as bioethics, the field is more associated with topics like cloning, stem cell research, neuroscience, and genetic engineering than with topics in ordinary medical care. Bioethics meetings devote as much time—and journals as much space—to discussions of speculative science as they do to discussions of medical practice. Although a significant number of people continue to concentrate on clinical ethics, the field as a whole seems preoccupied with cutting-edge science and medical innovation.

Societies and scholars should give serious thought to the ethical implications of scientific and medical advances, and we have all spent time teaching and writing about such advances. Nevertheless, we are more certain than ever that the everyday problems of patients and clinicians deserve serious consideration. Indeed, in today's medical environment, bedside ethics is as important as it has ever been. Too many clinicians lack the skill, opportunity, or will to have the difficult conversations that help patients and families cope with serious illness. Busy doctors don't have time to discuss much of anything with patients, partly because insurance plans pay them more for performing procedures than for talking with patients. And, we live in a culture that continues to treat illness and death as alien events, leaving patients and families to struggle through largely on their own.

This book is our effort to renew attention to the ethical problems faced by seriously ill patients and their caregivers. Some of the most meaningful contributions to medical ethics have come from writers Art Frank calls "humanistic reformers." In their perceptive accounts of interactions between patients and doctors, Jay Katz and Eric Cassell gave readers a real sense of what can go right and wrong in medical care.[2] We see ourselves continuing in this tradition, but with a more explicit focus on how patients and caregivers experience real-world ethics.

We hope to revitalize a medical ethics tradition that has lost some force over the years. Medical ethics is a diverse and wide-ranging field, covering everything from the most abstract analysis of deontological moral theory to a nuts-and-bolts discussion of how to make a living will. The field has room for many voices, and we think first-person accounts of serious illness belong in the medical ethics conversation.

PERSONAL STORIES AND ETHICS:
THE CONNECTIONS

We believe that the experiences and reflections of patients and caregivers should inform and guide ethical judgments in medicine. As the saying goes, "good ethics start with good facts." Our stories contain information about what it is like to be a patient in today's health care system and what it is like to be the family caregiver for such a patient. Our stories also show how standard ethical principles like respecting patient autonomy and protecting patients' interests operate in the real world.

We present our stories and reflections as ethical observers. Our experiences led us to see ethical dimensions of patient care that we hadn't appreciated before. In our medical ethics work, we are accustomed to having doctors and students tell us that none of their recent cases raised interesting ethical issues. Yet, when we ask them to describe a few of those cases, we invariably find much to discuss. Part of the medical ethicist's job is to point to assumptions, judgments, and actions that raise ethical issues. So, it's not surprising that once we became the subjects of medical cases, we discovered ethical issues we hadn't recognized earlier. Personal experience led most of us to expand our view of what counts as ethical in the illness experience.

We use stories to justify ethical claims, too. We make ethical judgments and draw ethical conclusions. We describe behavior we believe was morally praiseworthy, as well as behavior that patients and caregivers should not have to deal with. We describe ethical gray areas, too—places where we disagree or aren't sure about the right thing to do. We expect readers to question or disagree with our judgments, and we encourage them to share their views. We want to provoke more conversation and thought about the ethics of serious illness. We believe there is still much to learn about ethics in patient care.

We also think detailed personal stories like ours can enrich and supplement the case-based approach to medical ethics. In the typical case presentation, doctors give a relatively brief account of a particular patient's situation and the issues arising in that patient's care. But such accounts leave out information that should be part of the ethical analysis. In the standard case presentation, for example, no one reports how much time the doctor spent explaining the patient's diagnosis and treatment options. No one reports whether the doctor made eye contact while greeting the patient or took seriously the patient's complaints about side effects. Although these "constant, small ethical decisions of everyday clinical work"[3] have a significant impact on patients and care-givers, they are usually overlooked in ethics analysis.

Another shortcoming of the conventional case-based approach is that it reflects the clinician's view of the patient's circumstances. This view will often be inadequate, for clinicians may fail to grasp significant elements of the case. As Leon Kass remarked at one of our meetings, "Without a good understanding of what it is like to be overwhelmed by the experience of illness—one's own or that of a loved one—how can the doctor or ethicist appreciate the human situation the doctor must address?" Our stories are written from perspectives often missing from standard ethics cases. We present a different view of "the facts" than the doctors involved in our care would present.

TOWARD A PATIENT-CENTERED ETHICS

As patients and caregivers, we learned about the distance between medical ethics in books and classrooms, and medical ethics on the ground. It is one thing to teach students about the elements of informed consent; it's another thing to be a seriously ill patient making a complicated treatment decision with uncertain outcomes. It is one thing to read about our overtaxed health care system, it's another thing to put your life in the hands of that system.

We hold members of our own field—including ourselves—responsible for some of the problems we encountered as patients and caregivers. Critics argue that the increased presence of medical ethicists in schools and hospitals hasn't done much to improve how patients are treated. According to the critics, the field has not done enough to promote a more patient-centered approach to medical care.

We think there is some validity to this charge. For example, in teaching about patient autonomy, medical ethicists have left too many doctors with the impression that they should refrain from making recommendations or raising questions about the choices patients make. Too many doctors think they must remain silent once their patient makes a treatment choice, even if they think that choice is unwise. Patients are no better off with this sort of abandonment than they were with old-style medical paternalism. Ethicists also haven't done enough to discourage the checklist approach to informed consent, in which clinicians recite boilerplate information about treatment options and make little effort to determine whether patients understand the material they have heard. This approach obviously doesn't give patients a real opportunity to participate in decisions about their care.

Another problem is that medical ethics too rarely incorporates personal perspectives on illness. People in our field haven't given adequate consideration to what patients and families think about the practices and issues that are the focus of our work. The typical medical ethics analysis evaluates problems from the clinician's perspective. This is understandable, for most medical ethicists work in academic institutions and hospitals. Much of our teaching and writing is intended to help clinicians and students respond to the ethical issues they confront in their work. Yet, adopting the clinician perspective can limit and distort our view of the ethical situation, which can in turn reduce the value of our judgments and recommendations.

As patients and caregivers, we saw ethical issues from a new vantage point. An example comes from my own experience. Before becoming a cancer patient, I had spent many years teaching medical students about ethics and gifts from patients to doctors. In these sessions, I emphasized the potential negative effects of accepting gifts. Gifts can impair the doctor's professional judgment, which can have a variety of bad consequences for patients.

But, as a patient, I became more aware of gift-giving's positive effects. One day, as my partner Peter Joy and I drove to a doctor appointment, he pulled out a package he was planning to give the doctor. This doctor was a favorite of Peter's, and the two had discovered a mutual liking for an offbeat brand of ties. Unbeknownst to me, Peter had bought one of these ties for the doctor. I realized that this was a sincere and generous gesture, a gesture I wasn't about to question. The doctor was surprised and pleased when Peter presented the gift. It was a nice moment amidst the abundant bad moments we had had together. The experience taught me how meaningful and restorative gift-giving can be for patients and their families. I still think it's important to consider the potential harm that gift-giving can create, but I now have a deeper understanding of its benefits.

Besides paying more attention to how patients and families see ethical issues, a patient-centered medical ethics would consider how illness is experienced in the wider social world. It is difficult to find ethics material that even mentions what happens to patients and caregivers when they are away from the medical setting. Yet, sick people regularly encounter inappropriate and thoughtless behavior by individuals they meet in everyday life. Indeed, memoirs by patients and families are depressingly full of stories about the damage such behavior inflicts.

An example comes from Marjorie Williams, who was in her forties when she was diagnosed with terminal liver cancer. Williams described how furious she became "any time someone tried to cheer me up by reciting the happy tale of a sister-in-law's cousin who had liver cancer but now he's eighty and he hasn't been troubled by it in forty years." Williams wrote, "I was working so hard to accept my death: I felt abandoned, evaded, when someone insisted I would live."[4]

For patients, false hope is usually more toxic than therapeutic. Remarks like the one Williams described may be intended to help patients, but in reality can have the opposite effect. We wonder why people in our field haven't given more thought to the harm inflicted by this sort of behavior. After what we have gone through, it seems obvious that our profession ought to consider how friends and acquaintances can act and speak ethically in the presence of someone coping with serious illness. As we dealt with cancer, we came into contact with quite a few people whose efforts to provide comfort went awry. *New York Times* critic Janet Maslin said it well: "A sick or dying person should not have to deal with lies, competitiveness, or an exaggerated sense of catastrophe. Yet the speaker unaccustomed to empathy will have no better idea of what to say."[5] Medical ethics is one field that could help with this societal deficit.

MUNDANE MEDICAL HARMS

We write about many good things that happened to us as patients and caregivers, but we also describe things that should not have happened. Earlier chapters recount some of our good and bad experiences, but there are others worth noting.

We begin with the negatives. Now that we have been patients and caregivers, we see ethical problems that we didn't fully recognize before. Our expectations of how certain matters would be handled were at times inaccurate. In retrospect, we can see that we were naïve about many dimensions of serious illness.

Some of our difficulties can be traced to institutional rules and customs—what Art Frank refers to as "the mundane ways in which clinical practice sacrifices generous care to organizational necessity." In reporting our difficulties, we join many other patients and caregivers who have written about this sort of harm. We can only hope that our "insider" status will add weight to their claims. The problems we describe are both real and in need of remedy.

We now have first-hand knowledge of some of the harms produced by institutional timetables. While we were ill, several of us needed care on weekends or holidays. But cancer centers and doctors' offices are usually closed at those times. When we had disturbing symptoms during off hours, we had to choose between two bad options. We could go to the emergency room and wait—typically for hours—until someone could see us and decide whether our problems were serious. Or, we could grin and bear it, hoping we would be all right until the next regular workday. Work schedules can produce painful delays for grieving families, too. The Memorial Day backlog at the medical examiner's office extended John Robertson's terrible wait for his beloved wife's ashes.

We would be the first to argue that health care and morgue workers deserve respite from their difficult duties. But illness and death don't operate according to the standard work week. Wouldn't it be possible to stagger time off, so that patients and families could get the services they need? In a welcome development, cancer centers are beginning to establish special twenty-four-hour emergency rooms for their patients. Innovations like this could go a long way toward easing cancer's burdens.

There were also times when our medical care did not go the way it should have gone. In our group, the most serious missteps involved the cancer diagnosis. When doctors overlook or misinterpret signs of cancer, patients pay the price. With advanced disease, survival odds go down, and treatment becomes more brutal. Anger, anxiety, and a sense of betrayal are the emotional by-products of delayed diagnosis. When doctors fail to make a timely diagnosis, it becomes hard for patients and families to trust the medical system.

Most of the problems with our care were less serious, but they still had bad consequences. Here are a few of the mishaps that occurred. Worried family members were told that a patient's tumor was benign, when in fact it was malignant. Hospital patients' calls for help went unanswered until relatives intervened. Cancer center staff lost track of patients waiting for chemotherapy, making long days even longer. Busy residents neglected to set up appointments and procedures they had promised to arrange. Records were misplaced, phone messages overlooked, and e-mails unanswered.

There were other incidents that should have gone differently. Doctors conducted what should have been private conversations in crowded waiting rooms. Patients were given a controversial anti-anemia drug without being informed of its risks and questionable effectiveness in cancer patients.[6] Clinicians failed to warn of the depression that often occurs after cancer treatment ends, when medical attention diminishes and patients wait for the tests that will show whether the treatment was effective. Hospice workers seemed to put ideology above patient comfort, refusing to permit intravenous pain medications for a dying patient.

We realize that problems like those we encountered are to be expected in complex institutions like modern hospitals and cancer centers. Most of the time, we put up with the glitches without making a fuss. Yet, they did take a toll. It would be wonderful if patients and families could be spared the added burdens imposed by disturbing events like these.

Last, but not least, were the painful reminders that communication skills are not a prerequisite for earning a medical degree. Most of us have vivid memories of startling and unnerving remarks by clinicians involved in our care. For example, a prominent specialist talking with Art Frank about test results muttered, "It's either primary or secondary tumors. I'll send a report to your doctor." That was it—no expression of concern, no offer to take questions. The message Art received was, "Get out of my lab. I don't want you here."[7] On the telephone, a cheerful radiologist confirming Patty Marshall's breast cancer diagnosis told her she shouldn't worry too much about her "regular, garden-variety" breast cancer. Later, after Patty had been through two surgeries and was preparing to undergo weeks of chemotherapy and radiation treatments, another annoyingly perky doctor—someone Patty described as "so chipper, so healthy, so unaffected by life's torments"—used up valuable appointment time urging Patty to take up long-distance running. Weakened and in pain at that point, Patty was finding it hard just to make it through the day.

These were just a few of the times when doctors seemed unaware of the impact their words would have on us. We understand how this can happen. For the doctors, it was just another day at work. Talking to cancer patients was nothing special; it was simply part of their everyday routine. Meanwhile, like most people dealing with cancer, we were scared and on-edge, filled with a sense of impending disaster. When clueless clinicians made off-hand or dismissive remarks, we felt terrified or abandoned.

Because patients often lack the presence of mind—or the courage—to react openly to such remarks, clinicians may never learn of the distress they have created. Our best doctors and nurses remained alert to their patients' precarious state of mind. We wish all clinicians would remember to choose their words carefully when talking with seriously ill patients.

PRICELESS BENEFITS

There were times when we were disappointed by the medical system, but also times when the opposite was true. Of course, those of us still standing are immensely grateful for the treatment that has kept us going. For the most part, the care we received was competent, and some of it was better than that. Most of the clinicians we encountered were reasonably good at their work. Many doctors and nurses were able to be both professional and empathetic as they helped us through treatment. The oncology nurses were particularly impressive—efficient but not brusque, upbeat but not saccharine, sympathetic but not cloying. We owe a lot to these dedicated women and men who labor long and hard for relatively modest wages.

We also had doctors who went above and beyond the call of duty. Some doctors shared their own illness stories with us. Some were quite good at explaining our options and helping us figure out what we wanted to do. Some arranged for us to speak with other doctors who could provide second opinions on how to proceed. Some showed extraordinary concern for our physical and emotional well-being. Some praised our strength and admired our courage as we suffered through our ordeals.

Certain doctors were also able to forge meaningful connections with patients facing a dire prognosis. They did simple things like sit quietly in a patient's darkened hospital room or compliment a patient's choice in eyeglasses. These doctors gave us enormous comfort by responding not only to our medical needs, but to our needs as persons dealing with life-threatening illness.

Ethical medical care involves minimizing harm and maximizing benefit to patients. It involves treating patients with respect and dignity. These principles apply not just to the most significant ethical matters like end-of-life care, but also to smaller matters like waiting times in doctors' offices and promises to call in prescriptions.[8] Our cancer experiences taught us how important the smaller matters can be. We don't think it would take much to fix some of the problems we describe, nor do we think it would be very hard for clinicians to do more of the things that meant so much to us as patients and caregivers.

COMPLEXITIES AND PUZZLES

We've written about ways that both clinicians and ordinary people can help individuals coping with cancer. We've described words and actions we believe would be welcomed by most patients and caregivers. But we also recognize that the same responses won't work for everyone. Not every patient wants an in-depth discussion of her illness and the future. Some patients prefer not to know the precise odds for treatment success (and failure). Some need rosy generalizations, while others do better with cold, hard facts. And individuals are not the same at every visit. Sometimes even the hard-nosed realist needs a dose of optimism to get through the day.

In the course of our conversations, we learned that our cancer responses were far from identical. Some of the variation can be attributed to the different sorts of cancer, cancer treatments, and cancer outcomes we experienced. But some of the variation reflected the different life experiences we brought to cancer. As Eric Cassell has written, "Life experiences—previous illness, experiences with doctors, hospitals, medications, deformities and disabilities, pleasures and successes, or miseries and failures—form the background for illness."[9]

The ways we thought about cancer depended partly on our personal illness histories. Several of us have cancer in our families, and some have watched close relatives die of cancer. Some of us are, in Art Frank's words, "twofers or threefers" who have weathered more than one health crisis in a relatively short time. Art himself had a heart attack the year before his cancer diagnosis, and his mother-in-law died of cancer about a year after he went through cancer treatment. Patty Marshall was just beginning to bounce back from her cancer when her husband was diagnosed with the cancer that ended his life just a few weeks later. As Patty described it, "In a one-year period, I felt like I got hit and hit and hit and hit." Dan Brock and Norm Fost have a relatively matter-of-fact attitude toward their cancers, partly because they have dealt with other, more serious illnesses. Cancer is "the Big C" for most of us, but for them, as Dan put it, cancer is "a little c" while they both face "a big something else."

In short, cancer was different for each of us, and this affected our needs as patients and caregivers. Some of us were more shocked than others when cancer appeared. Some were more overwhelmed than others. Some needed more support than others. Besides the variation among individuals, there was variation within individuals. Each of us needed different things at different times. Sometimes we appreciated sympathy, but other times we resented it. Sometimes we wanted lots of attention, but sometimes we wanted to be left alone.

Our conversations about individual variation brought home the complexity of the doctor's task. What each of us wanted and needed from our doctors depended in part on what we brought to cancer. How could the doctors know our specific backgrounds and preferences? How could they know whether to present a general or a detailed picture of what we were facing? How could they know whether to be upbeat or dispassionate in discussing our prospects? How could they know what sort of reassurance would work best for us? How could they know what we needed on that particular day?

As a result of our discussions, we have a better understanding of the difficulties doctors face. Even after a long and close relationship with a cancer patient, the spouses in our group learned that "it's hard to be there in the right way."[10] It is unrealistic to expect doctors and other clinicians to be precisely attuned to the specific needs of a seriously ill patient they have met only recently.

Although we should not expect perfection from our doctors, we do think it's fair to expect some sensitivity. Good clinicians know how to find out about a patient's particular mindset. They know how to watch and listen, question and probe. The best doctors ask direct questions to determine whether patients prefer details or generalities. They ask open-ended questions that give patients an opportunity to reveal their fears, desires, and priorities. They bring up matters that most patients worry about, like problems that come up during cancer treatment and how long it takes to recover from them. And they bring up these topics without waiting for individual patients to ask about them. As we learned, not asking is not equivalent to not wanting to know. Patients may be silent because they do not know what to ask or do not want to take up too much of the doctor's time. Good doctors bring up common concerns and give individual patients a chance to invite or decline further discussion.

Our group discussions made us more aware of individual differences among patients and the difficulties such differences create for doctors. We also unearthed a few ethical questions that were difficult to settle. Certain situations left us puzzled about the best way to proceed. Perhaps the biggest puzzle was how to handle suspicious test findings.

In "Learning the Bad News," John Robertson describes the harm that can come when doctors evade their responsibilities to tell patients about a cancer diagnosis. But what should happen when the evidence of cancer is unclear? The puzzle arises when a scan or other test reveals the possible presence of cancer. Ambiguous test results can be the first step to a cancer diagnosis; for patients who have had cancer before, ambiguous results can signal a possible recurrence or a new cancer. But more tests will be necessary to determine whether the initial finding signifies cancer. When doctors ask patients to return for further testing, what reason should they give? Should doctors acknowledge that cancer is a possibility? Should they do so only when a patient seeks an explanation for the additional testing? Or, should doctors be more forthcoming than that, since many patients who suspect cancer will be too frightened to raise the issue?

These questions emerged in our conversations about diagnosis and follow-up examinations. Dan Brock recalled a long-ago incident in which he was asked to return for further testing after a routine eye examination. When Dan asked why, the ophthalmologist replied that the exam had uncovered an abnormality in Dan's vision. The doctor said it probably wasn't anything serious, but he needed more information before he could be sure of that. After Dan pressed for more details, the doctor declared, "You might have a brain tumor." Dan endured a week of high anxiety until the next round of tests showed that he was fine.

Dan was not happy with the way his doctor handled this suspicious finding. For years, he considered it a classic example of a premature and unnecessarily harmful disclosure. But, as we exchanged stories about suspicious findings, he became less certain that his doctor had done the wrong thing.

One of my experiences illustrates the difficulty in determining right and wrong in this situation. In my case, I learned about a suspicious spot on one of my follow-up scans a full year after it was detected. My doctors had been watching to see whether the spot appeared larger in subsequent scans. If it stayed the same size for two years, they could safely conclude it wasn't a tumor. When one of my doctors finally mentioned the spot, I was disturbed that no one had told me about it earlier. If it had turned out to be cancerous, I think I would have been angry that I had been kept in the dark for a year. Yet, I was also disturbed that I would have to wait another year to find out whether this was a true or false alarm. A part of me wished that no one had told me about the spot. It would have been nice to remain blissfully ignorant of this particular suspicious finding.

As this incident suggests, I'm not sure whether I want to hear about suspicious findings right away, or only after follow-up tests show that the situation is truly serious. Some patients have a definite preference, but the preferences go in either direction. As Norm Fost pointed out, "patients are idiosyncratic. Some want everything. Some want nothing. Short of saying something like, 'I know something you don't know,' it's hard [for the doctor] to know the right thing to do." When doctors follow cancer patients over the long term, they can ask patients whether they prefer early or late disclosure. But this strategy isn't available to doctors seeing patients for the first time. And some patients, like me, will have a hard time figuring out their preferences.

The bottom line is that suspicious findings present a no-win situation for patients. On one hand, immediate disclosure can generate high anxiety before there is a real basis for concern. On the other hand, doctors who fail to disclose suspicious findings deny patients an opportunity to prepare for the possibility that they have cancer. We weren't able to settle on a satisfactory resolution to the disclosure problem. From the patient's perspective, suspicious findings are bad news no matter when they are disclosed.

LARGER LESSONS

Cancer showed us specific ways to put ethical principles into practice, but many of its lessons were more far-reaching. Facing serious illness was something most of us had never done before. Blessed with reasonably good health, our previous medical choices had been relatively simple. Cancer altered our thinking about medical care.

Before cancer, most of us were unfamiliar with the psychological impact of serious illness. Now we know that cancer patients and caregivers operate in crisis mode. There is the shock of the diagnosis, there is confusion about what to do, there is the sense that mortality is just around the corner. Once in these circumstances, we learned that medical decision-making was harder than we had expected.

Having cancer also taught us how much we were willing to sacrifice for the chance to live longer. Before becoming patients and caregivers, most of us had spent years teaching, thinking, and writing about life-sustaining treatment for seriously ill patients. We were quite familiar with the burdens and side effects of cancer treatments, and we knew that brutal treatment regimens were often ineffective. Before we became cancer patients and caregivers, we had more doubts about the value of aggressive cancer treatments than many people have.

We may have been relatively skeptical about cancer treatments, but that did not stop us from wanting them. Survival was our paramount objective. Several of us endured burdensome chemotherapy and radiation regimens to maximize our chances for survival. We also accepted higher risks of long-lasting side effects in exchange for better survival odds. We made those decisions without much hesitation. When we were facing life-threatening cancer, quality of life seemed less important than it once did.

That doesn't mean we have become vitalists—people who believe in sustaining life at any cost. Indeed, we now have a better idea of when we would call a halt to treatment. Yet, as Dan explains in his chapter on questionable-benefit treatments, we have also developed a better understanding of why patients, families, and doctors pursue treatments that seem unjustified to outside observers. When medicine offers people a chance at longer life, most people are likely to want that chance.

In life-and-death situations, patients and families often want to try interventions that seem excessive and unreasonable to others. We don't believe that clinicians must always provide interventions in those circumstances, but we also don't believe that frustration and anger are the right ways to respond. Until you are face-to-face with death, you cannot appreciate how difficult it is to let go of life. Even when patients and families agree not to pursue life-sustaining treatment, "dying still stings."[11] Patients and families who have a hard time giving up on treatment ought to receive compassion and emotional support, not hostility.

The strength of the survival urge can lead patients to make unanticipated choices, too. Some of us learned first-hand how treatment preferences can change with the advent of serious illness. The most striking change came when Patty Marshall's husband, Larry Heinrich, was diagnosed with the cancer that ended his life. Ten years earlier, he had undergone chemotherapy and radiation for a different form of cancer. Once that treatment was over, he insisted he would never again go through such an ordeal. Yet, when the second cancer was discovered, Larry wanted to try chemotherapy. He chose to try this intervention even though the best it could offer was a few more weeks of life.

Everyone should be aware that their ideas about acceptable and unacceptable treatment might change once they face a real medical crisis. Change can go in either direction. People who think they would reject certain interventions may later find reasons to accept them. Some of us were surprised at what we were willing to endure in exchange for a better chance at life. People who insist they want "everything done" can change their minds, too. For example, at first John's wife, Carlota, wanted every available cancer therapy. Near the end of her life, however, she decided against having the last-resort measure she was offered. Our medical ethics colleague Susan Wolf has written of her father's similar change of heart. As his cancer got worse, her father switched "from a lifetime of 'spare no effort'" to a choice to cease all life-sustaining measures.[12] These examples show that treatment preferences are fluid, not fixed. As circumstances change, patients' decisions may change as well.

Cancer also teaches grim lessons about the limits of our control. Before cancer, we went through life with some sense that we were in charge. At an intellectual level, we knew that this was an illusion. We had only to glance at the headlines to see how nature, war, and human behavior disrupt individual plans and lives on an everyday basis. But it was cancer that revealed the true limits of our power. Cancer revealed that we were, like everyone else, "at the mercy of the accidents of things."[13]

With cancer, we learned that our fates would be determined largely by forces beyond our control. Our own bodies were out of control; that is why we had the tumors that threatened our lives. We couldn't control whether the tumors would respond to treatment. We couldn't control whether we would have treatment side effects and complications. If we were lucky enough to go into remission, we couldn't control how long it would last.

Much of what happened to us in the medical system was beyond our control, too. We could choose our doctors, but those choices were constrained by practical considerations like where we lived. We could choose which treatments to have, but those options were limited, as well. Cancer grants patients just a small space in which to exercise choice and control. Biology and other fortuities determine most of what happens to patients.

Our relative helplessness had carry-over effects. We were all professors, accustomed to speaking our minds. Yet, with cancer, even the boldest among us became meek. Norm Fost spoke of the powerful "desire to be a good patient" and of "not wanting to annoy the doctor." Some of us were surprised at how passive we became. We usually did what doctors and nurses told us to do. More often than not, we *wanted* them to tell us what to do. Deprived of our usual self-confidence, we weren't sure how to operate in this new cancer world. Most of us needed more direction than we would have expected.

We could not control our fates, but hoped passionately for life. It was a tense situation. During treatment, we concentrated on immediate challenges like getting dressed every day and getting to chemotherapy on time. The rest of the time, however, we hoped and we worried. We knew the statistics on treatment outcomes, but we didn't know where we would end up. In waiting rooms and chemotherapy suites, we gazed at other patients and wondered which of us would be alive next year. Some patients had to end up in the group that didn't survive—would it be them or us?

Cancer brought home the limits of our power, leaving us sadder, but wiser, about life. We are deeply aware that life-threatening illness operates according to its own rules, and we know that, as Patty Marshall put it, "we do not choose our time." We know we can't count on doing everything we want to do, finishing every project we want to finish, spending as much time with loved ones as we want to spend. We have been, in Leon Kass's words, "shaken out of the complacency of our own plans and our belief that our lives are ours to design and will go on forever." And we have learned that, in Patty's words, "some things are not that important." It is sobering, but also liberating, to know these things. If it weren't for cancer, we wouldn't know them as well as we do.

Cancer was a test of personal character, too. We aren't fond of the military metaphors that have generated so many cancer clichés—references to cancer wars, fights, battles, and so forth—but we did feel we were engaged in a struggle. Getting through cancer required strength, perseverance, and stoicism. Cancer took us away from work and treasured pastimes. We couldn't do things like teach, travel, run, or hike in the woods. We tried to accept cancer's burdens and constraints with grace and dignity, but it wasn't easy. We were proud and independent people who suddenly felt weak and vulnerable. We muddled through, sometimes rising to the occasion, sometimes, as Art Frank put it, being dragged to the occasion. As I said earlier, we didn't feel that we had a lot of control over what was happening to us.

Sometimes it seemed unfair that cancer had singled us out. We knew well the objective facts: Millions are diagnosed with cancer every year, and there was no reason why we shouldn't be among them. Nevertheless, we weren't immune from asking the "why me?" question. Did we do something to deserve this affliction? Was cancer some kind of payback for thinking that we knew something about serious illness and morality? We do not think the world works that way, but have to admit that every once in a while we did feel victimized.

Although it sometimes seemed unfair that we were the ones facing cancer, cancer also brought constant reminders of our privileged positions. Not only did we have personal connections to experts who could help us with medical matters, we had good jobs and good health care coverage.[14] We could take time off from work without putting our jobs in jeopardy. Nearly all of the shockingly high costs of our treatment and follow-up care would be paid by our health plans. We weren't at risk of losing coverage or being denied reimbursement for expensive procedures. We did not have to worry about being fired or going bankrupt because of cancer.

We are exceedingly thankful to have escaped cancer's financial burdens. We came into contact with others who were not so fortunate. During chemotherapy, I overheard one breast cancer patient telling a nurse that she needed to cancel her next appointment. The patient said she had used up her sick leave and would lose her job as a security guard if she missed another day of work. Patty Marshall knew a woman who was a financially comfortable postal worker when she was diagnosed with breast cancer. Because she couldn't keep working after she become ill, her once middle-class family descended into poverty.

When we faced cancer, we took advantage of our connections, generous health coverage, and insider knowledge. We did so with some guilt, but not much hesitation. Our feelings were similar to those of Marjorie Williams, another cancer patient with advantages like ours. Williams recognized the unfairness inherent in her privileged position, but also observed, "when your own time comes, you will pull pretty much every string available to get what you need."[15] Perhaps we should have refrained from some of our string-pulling, but it was hard to see how that would have done other patients much good.

Although we took the opportunities that were available to us, we abhor the current disparities in cancer care. Before cancer, we were advocates for a more equitable health care system; after cancer, we are even more disturbed by the inequities. Cancer patients need a better safety net than the one that now exists. Every cancer patient should have access to a reasonable level of care. Loss of livelihood should not be part of the price cancer exacts. Take it from us: Cancer alone is more than enough for patients and families to handle.

Cancer taught us about the complexities of treatment decision-making. Cancer showed us how health care inequality plays out in the real world. Cancer exposed the limits of our power and control. Cancer laid bare our dependence on others. Cancer revealed what—and who—we really care about. Valuable lessons, though painful to learn.

CLOSING THOUGHTS

Throughout this book, we make recommendations that could improve the lives of cancer patients and caregivers. Many of the recommendations seem obvious. For example, everyone knows that doctors should make sure cancer patients understand the consequences of their treatment choices. Everyone knows that friends should offer support when someone close to them has cancer. But, as we discovered, people don't always practice what they know. There is a gap between cancer ideals and cancer actions.

Moreover, it wasn't clear to us that "everyone" knows how to behave ethically toward seriously ill patients and their families. A surprising number of people said things that made us feel worse, not better. Then there were the ones who avoided us altogether. Did they think that avoiding us would make the cancer go away? We don't know whether they were unable or simply unwilling to get in touch, but we do know that the lack of contact left us feeling lonely and stigmatized.

We hope our stories convince people to reach out when someone they know has cancer. We hope our stories teach people what helps and harms seriously ill patients and their families. We hope our stories persuade people to practice the ethics they know.

We cannot in good conscience end on a cheerful note. There are ways to make cancer less onerous, but there is no way to eliminate its burdens. Even when treatment is effective and the prognosis good, cancer leaves its scars. Some of cancer's scars are physical, but most are in the mind.

For most of us, cancer was the first real notice of our mortality. Cancer cut through the social and biological programming that keeps death at a distance. People diagnosed with cancer no longer see death as something that happens to others. Loved ones caring for patients get this message second-hand, but more forcefully than ever before.

Cancer revealed how foolish we were in thinking we were prepared for life-threatening illness. Cancer made us realize how hard it will be to let go of the people we love and the work that gives our lives meaning. Cancer showed us that, even when death is the most merciful outcome, death is never a good outcome.

We offer some reassurance and some hope for lessening cancer's burdens. With the help of many wonderful people, we did get through cancer. And we gained some wisdom in the process. But we refuse to be upbeat about cancer. Cancer tested our character and our relationships. Dealing with cancer was hard work, and we didn't always do it well. Cancer is surely instructive, but its teachings can break your heart.

Notes

1. In our discussion, John Robertson labeled these matters "important but not interesting" to scholars in the field.
2. Jay Katz, *The Silent World of Doctor and Patient* (New Haven: Yale University Press, 1984, 2nd ed. 2002); Eric Cassell, *The Nature of Suffering and the Goals of Medicine* (New York: Oxford University Press, 1991, 2nd ed. 2004).
3. Art Frank, transcript.
4. Marjorie Williams, "Hit By Lightening," in *The Woman at the Washington Zoo: Writings on Politics, Family, and Fate*, ed. Timothy Noah (New York: PublicAffairs, 2005), 335.
5. Janet Maslin, "Open Mouth, Remove Boorishness: A Guide," *New York Times*, December 19, 2005.
6. The FDA has a new program intended to address this problem. See Mike Mitka, "New Oversight Put in Place for Physicians Giving Anemia Drugs to Patients With Cancer," *JAMA* 303 (2010): 1355–56.
7. The quotations are from a "found poem" that is based on an interview with Art. See Loreen Herwaldt, *Patient Listening: A Doctor's Guide* (Iowa City: University of Iowa Press, 2008), 38.
8. For more on "smaller matter" ethics, see Rebecca Dresser, "Dignity and the Seriously Ill Patient," in *Human Dignity and Bioethics* (Washington, DC: President's Council on Bioethics, 2008), 505–12. Retrieved from http://bioethics.georgetown.edu/pcbe/index.html
9. Cassell, *Nature of Suffering*, 37.
10. Patty Marshall, transcript.
11. Greg Sachs, "Sometimes Dying Still Stings," *JAMA* 284 (2000): 2423.
12. Susan M. Wolf, "Confronting Physician-Assisted Suicide and Euthanasia: My Father's Death," *Hastings Center Report* 38, no. 5 (2008): 23–36.
13. Leon Kass, transcript.
14. Art Frank's sense of privilege is different from others in our group, for he lives in Canada and was treated there. Art received the same "generic care" that anyone living in his province would have received at the time. But compared with what was available in other parts of the world, he says, that care was very good. As Art put it, "On the one hand, it's utterly democratic and on the other hand, it's completely privileged."
15. Williams, *The Woman*, 324–25.

Index